MCQs for the Final FRCA

A 13. **A.** true **B.** false **C.** true **D.** false **E.** false

The Shrader probe is similar for all gases. The gas specific feature is the diameter of the collar, which is specific to fit the wall socket. The pipeline pressure is 400 kPa. The wall socket includes a seal to block the flow of gas when the probe is removed. After maintenance the line should be tested for both oxygen and nitrous oxide.

The British standard states that the probe should not twist while in the wall outlet. To prevent this the collar has a notch. The socket has a spring loaded outer ring. When this is depressed the probe is released and ejected.

A 14. **A.** false **B.** true **C.** false **D.** false **E.** true

Sevoflurane, carbon dioxide and nitrous oxide are known cerebrovascular vasodilators. They will increase regional blood flow and regional blood volume and hence raise intracranial pressure.

A 15. **A.** false **B.** false **C.** false **D.** true **E.** false

The right lung has two fissures. The oblique fissure separates the middle lobe from the lower lobe. It follows a line from the second vertebral spine to the sixth costochondral junction. The horizontal (transverse) fissure separates the upper lobe from the middle lobe. It follows a line from the fourth costochondral junction to join the oblique fissure in the axillary line.

Relationships of the right lung: Apex – extends into the root of the neck. The suprapleural membrane and pleural cupola are superior. The subclavian artery leaves a groove on the mediastinal surface of the lung.

Other relationships on the right are:

- The superior vena cava
- Right atrium lies anterior to the hilum
- The azygos vein arches over it

The bronchopulmonary segments of the right lung are:

- Upper lobe: apical, posterior and anterior
- Middle lobe: lateral and medial
- Lower lobe: apical, medial basal (cardiac), anterior, lateral and posterior

A 16. A. false **B.** false **C.** false **D.** false **E.** false

Bispectral analysis (BiS) was developed using the clinical end points of sedation. It relates to the hypnotic components of anaesthesia with a variety of inhalational and intravenous anaesthetic agents. It has been tested and validated in randomised clinical trails. It indicates the potential for awareness and of relative overdoses of hypnotic drugs. It does not predict movement or haemodynamic responses to stimulation. It does not predict the exact moment when consciousness returns.

BiS values of 65 to 85 have been recommended for sedation and 40 to 65 for general anaesthesia. Below 40, cortical suppression will be present correlating with raw EEG traces of burst suppression.

The possibility of postoperative spontaneous recall (awareness) has been shown to be extremely low at BiS <50. Conversely wakefulness is to be expected when the BiS score is >90. Return to consciousness is highly unlikely at BiS <65. But this does not predict when consciousness will occur.

Limitations on its use include ketamine anaesthesia and pre-existing neurological disease. EMG activity from scalp muscles can contaminate and give a falsely high BiS score.

A 17. A. true **B.** false **C.** false **D.** true **E.** false

Abductor palsy (unilateral or bilateral) occurs with partial or incomplete injury of the recurrent laryngeal nerve on the same side or on both sides of the vocal cords. The affected cord(s) assumes an adducted position, as the abductors are more sensitive to injury than the adductors. Pure adductor palsy is not known to occur.

Abductor and adductor palsy (unilateral or bilateral) occurs with a complete transection of the recurrent laryngeal nerve, e.g. at thyroidectomy. Both abductors and adductors are affected. The vocal cords rest in the neutral mid-position.

Total paralysis of the cords, which includes paralysis of the cricothyroid muscles (the tensor of the vocal cords), results from damage to the external motor branches of the superior laryngeal nerves as well as paralysis of the abductors and adductors supplied by the recurrent laryngeal nerves.

A **18.** **A.** true **B.** false **C.** true **D.** true **E.** true

Breathing spontaneously. The volume is plotted on the horizontal axis. The zero point for volume is on the right corresponding to the FRC. The flow is plotted on the vertical axis. The inspiratory flow is plotted below the horizontal axis moving to the left as the volume increases. It drops to zero flow at the end of inspiration. This corresponds to the tidal volume on the horizontal axis. The expiratory flow is shown above the horizontal axis. Its shape is determined by the rate of passive deflation of the lung.

Normal lung compliance is 1.5 to 2.0 l/kPa (150 to 200 ml cmH_2O).

A **19.** **A.** false **B.** false **C.** true **D.** true **E.** true

The cause of post dialysis hypoxia is not clear. Shunt, water overload and acidosis can lead to hypoxia but are unlikely to be present after dialysis. Hypoxia is common after dialysis and is most significant in the period immediately post-dialysis.

Possible causes include:

- Intrapulmonary leukostasis due to compliment activation
- Microatelectasis
- Increased pH (Bohr effect)
- Metabolism of small amounts of acetate (4 mmol/l) in bicarbonate dialysate can lead to a loss of carbon dioxide, under ventilation and hence hypoxia

A **20.** **A.** true **B.** false **C.** true **D.** true **E.** true

The effect on carbon dioxide tension will depend on whether the acidosis or the alkalosis predominates.

Definitions of massive blood transfusion include a transfusion of 500 ml blood (10% of blood volume) in less than 10 min or the giving of the patient's total blood volume in less than 24 h. These highlight the side-effects of giving blood.

Warmed blood does not have the effect of cold blood in reducing body temperature and reducing myocardial contractility due to cold.

The myocardium will be affected as stored blood is acidotic and hypocalcaemic due to the added citrate, which stops coagulation.

Stored blood has a high serum potassium level. The potassium rises by up to 0.5 mmol/l per day – less with SAGM blood – to reach 5 to 10 mmol in 500 ml by 4 weeks. Acidosis, hypocalcaemia and hypothermia aggravate the effects of hyperkalaemia on the heart.

The oxygen dissociation curve is shifted to the right by a fall in pH meaning that the haemoglobin will release more oxygen at a higher tension than normal. Carbon dioxide tension is affected by tissue metabolism and respiration. Once the total blood volume has been given there are probably no circulating antibodies to red cells making cross match meaningless.

A 21. **A.** true **B.** false **C.** true **D.** true **E.** true

The causes of DIC include septicaemia due to gram negative infections, meningococcus and malaria; malignancy; haemolytic mismatched transfusion reactions; trauma especially burns; venomous animal bites especially snakes.

Obstetric causes include abruption and amniotic fluid embolism.

Acute promyelocytic leukaemia is linked to chromosome t(15;17) translocation. One presentation is bleeding, which is aggravated by treatment. Treatment breaks down blast cells. This leads to more clotting factors and platelets being consumed and a DIC.

Fulminating meningococcal septicaemia or Water-Friderichsen syndrome activates compliment leading to a DIC.

A 22. **A.** false **B.** false **C.** false **D.** true **E.** false

The main problem with trauma to the liver is bleeding.
The remaining liver is not diseased and it will provide all the functions required of the body. Recovery is rapid. The liver arteries are not end-arteries and blood will be supplied through the portal circulation.

A 23. **A.** false **B.** false **C.** true **D.** false **E.** false

Sympathetic stimulation causes vasodilatation. The muscles of the orbit are supplied by the third cranial nerve, except for the lateral rectus supplied by the sixth (abducens) cranial nerve and the superior oblique by the fourth (trochlear) cranial nerve.

The fifth cranial nerve carries sensation from the face and is motor to masseter muscle. Nystagmus is caused by dysfunction of the cerebellum.

A **24.** **A.** true **B.** true **C.** true **D.** true **E.** true

A **25.** **A.** true **B.** false ?T **C.** false **D.** false **E.** false

The effects of sympathetic stimulation lead to:

- Tachycardia and a rise in arterial blood pressure
- Redistribution of blood flow from splanchnic to cerebral and coronary circulation
- Sweating and dilatation of the pupils
- An increase in blood glucose concentration
- Increased glycolysis and gluconeogenesis
- Increase in cellular metabolism throughout the body
- Increase in mental alertness

A **26.** **A.** false **B.** true **C.** true **D.** false **E.** true

The original and the short form of the McGill pain questionnaire are multidimensional but they do not test specifically for depression.

BJA CEPD Review 2002; 2(1)

A **27.** **A.** true **B.** true **C.** true **D.** true **E.** true

The causes of sudden loss of consciousness in a pregnant woman include:

1. Obstetric causes

- Haemorrhage leading to hypotension
- Aorto-caval compression leading to a reduced cardiac output
- Eclamptic fit
- Amniotic fluid embolism
- Pulmonary embolism
- Severe sepsis
- Venous air embolism

2. Anaesthetic causes

- Epidural or infiltration LA toxicity
- Total spinal
- Respiratory depression from epidural opioids

3. Miscellaneous
- Epileptic fit
- Vaso-vagal attack
- Cerebral haemorrhage
- Cardiac disease

A 28. **A.** false **B.** true **C.** false **D.** false **E.** false

PEEP reduces the risk of embolised air entering the heart. It increases right atrial pressure (RAP) but reduces left atrial pressure so increasing the risk of pulmonary air embolism.

Fluid loading increases pulmonary artery pressure, reducing the site to heart pressure gradient.

In surgery carrying a high risk of venous air embolism a central venous line should be placed before the operation is commenced

BJA CEPD Review 2002; 2(2)

A 29. **A.** false **B.** true **C.** true **D.** false **E.** false

Local anaesthetics produce cerebral depression of inhibitory areas before excitatory area hence the agitation that precedes loss of consciousness with local anaesthetic toxicity.

Diazepam and propofol or thiopentone will control the agitation. It is important to ensure good oxygenation. Intravenous anaesthesia is not recommended in children as the circulation through the humerus is sufficient to bypass the veins compressed by the tourniquet.

A 30. **A.** false **B.** false **C.** true **D.** true **E.** false

Status epilepticus is defined as continuous seizure activity lasting for 30 min or more. Or intermittent seizure activity lasting 30 min or more during which consciousness is not regained.

Approximately 50% of cases occur in the absence of a previous history of epilepsy. Lothman divides the changes that occur in epilepsy into two phases.

Phase 1
The increased cerebral metabolic demand caused by abnormally discharging cerebral cells is satisfied by an increase in cerebral

blood flow and an increase in autonomic activity that results in an increased arterial blood pressure; increased blood glucose level, sweating, hyperpyrexia and salivation.

Phase 2
Starts after approximately 30 min of seizure activity. It is characterised by failure of cerebral autoregulation, decreased cerebral blood flow, an increase in intracranial pressure and systemic hypertension.

The essential principles of the emergency management are ABC.

Pharmacological therapy. There is no ideal drug but the first line of treatment now is lorazepam 0.1 mg/kg given at 2 mg/min iv. It has been shown to be more effective than diazepam.

Anaesthesia 2001; 56: 648–659

Answers

Question	A	B	C	D	E
1	F	F	T	F	T
2	T	F	T	T	T
3	F	T	F	F	T
4	F	F	F	F	F
5	T	T	F	T	F
6	T	T	F	T	T
7	T	F	F	F	T
8	F	T	F	F	F
9	F	T	T	T	T
10	F	T	T	F	T
11	F	F	T	F	T
12	F	T	F	T	F
13	T	F	T	F	F
14	F	T	F	F	T
15	F	F	F	T	F
16	F	F	F	F	F
17	T	F	F	T	F
18	T	F	T	T	T
19	F	F	T	T	T
20	T	F	T	T	T
21	T	F	T	T	T
22	F	F	F	T	F
23	F	F	T	F	F
24	T	T	T	T	T
25	T	F	F	F	F
26	F	T	T	F	T
27	T	T	T	T	T
28	F	T	F	F	F
29	F	T	T	F	F
30	F	F	T	T	F

Section 2 – Questions

Paper 1 Questions

Q 1. The likely complications of laparoscopy include:

A. pneumothorax
B. shoulder pain
C. gas embolism
D. aspiration
E. left bundle branch block

Q 2. The likely results in an elderly, dehydrated man, breathing room air with prolonged bowel obstruction include:

A. respiratory alkalosis
B. metabolic acidosis
C. hypoxaemia
D. uraemia
E. anaemia

Q 3. The following are observed in a patient with acute tubular necrosis:

A. normal blood creatinine and high blood urea
B. excretion of small amounts of highly concentrated urine
C. hyperkalaemia
D. progressive increase in central venous pressure
E. casts in the urine

Q 4. Platelet concentrates:

A. are viable for 2 weeks
B. must be filtered when administered
C. may cause significant histamine release
D. must be cross-matched
E. contain citrate

Q 5. Dopaminergic receptor blockers:

A. decrease gastric emptying
B. decrease renal blood flow
C. relieve motion sickness
D. are used as anti-arrhythmics
E. are used to treat Parkinson's disease

Q 6. Injections of vitamin B_{12} are appropriate for patients with anaemia due to:

A. Chron's disease
B. a Vegan's diet
C. epileptics on phenytoin
D. pregnancy
E. a gastrectomy

Q 7. The following are associated with aortic incompetence:

A. rheumatic arthritis
B. syphilis
C. Ankylosing spondylitis
D. Marfan's syndrome
E. AIDS

Q 8. Concerning fat embolism syndrome:

A. A petechial rash is essential for a certain diagnosis
B. A fall in haematocrit is characteristic
C. Mental changes may be due to hypoxia
D. There may be a pyrexia
E. It occurs more commonly in tibial fractures than femoral fractures

Q 9. Intraocular pressure is normally:

A. 1.0 to 2.0 kPa above atmospheric pressure
B. increased by hypercarbia
C. reduced by non-depolarising neuromuscular blocking drugs
D. reduced by enflurane
E. reduced by trimetaphan

Q 10. Pulmonary surfactant:

- **A.** can be made synthetically
- **B.** is found in amniotic fluid at full term
- **C.** prevents alveolar collapse at low pressure
- **D.** is made by type 1 pneumocytes
- **E.** is a glycoprotein

Q 11. A maxillary nerve block in the pterygopalatine fossa gives anaesthesia of the:

- **A.** upper molars
- **B.** upper incisors
- **C.** soft palate
- **D.** anterior two-thirds of the tongue
- **E.** anterior part of the nasal septum

Q 12. The following may contribute to acute renal failure following abdominal surgery:

- **A.** pre-existing upper respiratory tract infection
- **B.** an induction dose of gentamycin
- **C.** massive blood transfusion
- **D.** endotoxaemia
- **E.** obstructive jaundice

Q 13. Air embolism is especially dangerous in the presence of:

- **A.** atrial septal defect (ASD)
- **B.** ventricular septal defect (VSD)
- **C.** tetralogy of Fallot
- **D.** aortic stenosis
- **E.** coarctation of the aorta

Q 14. Bilateral hilar lymphadenopathy is a recognised feature of:

- **A.** pulmonary tuberculosis
- **B.** Hodgkin's disease
- **C.** erythema multiformis
- **D.** systemic lupus erythematosus (SLE)
- **E.** pneumoconiosis

Paper 1 Questions

Q 15. The following can be derived from the blood gas analyser:

- **A.** base excess
- **B.** pH
- **C.** PCO_2
- **D.** standard bicarbonate
- **E.** actual bicarbonate

Q 16. In a patient with a healthy heart transplant undergoing elective non-cardiac surgery:

- **A.** a resting heart rate of 50 beats/min is normal
- **B.** the cardiovascular response to laryngoscopy is absent
- **C.** atropine will cause a tachycardia
- **D.** isoprenaline is the chronotrope of choice
- **E.** anti-rejection therapy should be stopped preoperatively

Q 17. Low molecular weight heparin:

- **A.** activity is effectively measured by activated partial thromboplastin time (APTT)
- **B.** strongly binds to plasma proteins
- **C.** has a longer plasma half-life than a standard heparin
- **D.** has its effect reversed by an equivalent dose of protamine
- **E.** has a prolonged plasma clearance in patients with renal failure

Q 18. Intrinsic (auto) positive end expiratory pressure (PEEP):

- **A.** can be achieved by reversing the I:E ratio
- **B.** does not result in air trapping when compared to extrinsic PEEP
- **C.** can be easily monitored in ITU patients
- **D.** has the same effect as extrinsic PEEP on haemodynamic values
- **E.** requires an extra work of breathing to initiate a spontaneous breath

Q 19. The effects of ecstasy (3,4-methylene dioxymethamphetamine):

- **A.** are dose related
- **B.** include hyperpyrexia, hypercalcaemia and hyperkalaemia

C. are due to inhibition of 5-hydroxytryptamine (5-HT)
D. are due to drinking large amounts of water
E. include renal failure due to rhabdomyolysis

Q 20. The following arrest the heart in diastole:

A. hypercalcaemia
B. hyperkalaemia
C. acidosis
D. hypothermia
E. digitalis overdose

Q 21. Exposure to nitrous oxide 20% in oxygen for a prolonged time causes:

A. sedation
B. respiratory depression
C. abdominal distension
D. leukopenia
E. vitamin B_{12} deficiency

Q 22. A pregnant lady who had an accidental dural tap and presented with headache, photophobia and hyperaesthesia of both lower limbs would be most appropriately treated with:

A. reassurance and review in 2 h
B. neurosurgical consultation
C. emergency CT scan
D. epidural saline
E. epidural blood patch

Q 23. A likely complications of infraclavicular block of the brachial plexus is:

A. recurrent laryngeal nerve paralysis
B. pneumothorax
C. air embolism
D. phrenic nerve paralysis
E. haemopericardium

Paper 1 Questions

Q 24. Withdrawal of life support treatment in ITU is based on:

A. age
B. patient autism
C. acute physiology and chronic health evalution (APACHE) score
D. predictable treatment outcome
E. clinical decision

Q 25. Stimulation of the 5th cranial nerve during posterior fossa surgery can cause:

A. jaw jerk
B. facial muscle twitching
C. bradycardia
D. shoulder jerking
E. nystagmus

Q 26. Chronic alcohol intake is associated with:

A. malnutrition
B. mean corpuscular volume (MCV) of 90
C. decreased gastric motility
D. decreased stress response to surgery
E. increased serum albumin

Q 27. The appropriate drug treatment of acute bronchoconstriction in children includes:

A. isoprenaline
B. ketamine
C. adrenaline
D. sodium cromoglicate
E. atropine

Q 28. Complications of a coeliac plexus block include:

A. constipation
B. hypertension
C. urinary retention
D. headache
E. impotence

Q 29. A decrease in hypoxic response to ventilation is seen in:

- **A.** patients at high altitudes
- **B.** cyanotic heart disease
- **C.** awakening from halothane anaesthesia
- **D.** iv PCA (patient controlled analgesia)
- **E.** pulmonary fibrosis

Q 30. Myotonic dystrophy is associated with:

- **A.** sternomastoid muscle wasting
- **B.** diabetes mellitus
- **C.** frontal baldness
- **D.** thyroid adenomata
- **E.** myasthenia gravis

Q 31. Pulmonary artery shunting is seen in:

- **A.** tetralogy of Fallot
- **B.** atrial septal defect
- **C.** pulmonary stenosis
- **D.** ventricular septal defect
- **E.** coarctation of the aorta

Q 32. Hepatic encephalopathy is precipitated by:

- **A.** surgery
- **B.** constipation
- **C.** oral neomycin
- **D.** haemorrhage
- **E.** benzodiazepines

Q 33. Concerning interosseous injection:

- **A.** It is the route of choice in the resuscitation of small children
- **B.** Swelling around the needle is not a reason for discontinuation
- **C.** Aspiration of marrow confirms the position
- **D.** The humerus is preferable to other bones
- **E.** Only crystalloid can be given

Q 34. The following are used in the direct calculation of $P(A\text{-}a)O_2$:

- **A.** $C(a\text{-}v)O_2$
- **B.** oxygen delivery
- **C.** oxygen consumption
- **D.** alveolar nitrogen tension
- **E.** respiratory quotient

Q 35. Old age is associated with:

- **A.** an increased minimum alveolar concentration (MAC) value for volatile agents
- **B.** resistance to non-depolarising drugs
- **C.** a decreased functional residual capacity (FRC)
- **D.** sensitivity to morphine
- **E.** decreased autonomic function and efficiency

Q 36. The treatment of pre-eclampsia with magnesium sulphate administration is associated with:

- **A.** depression of cardiac output
- **B.** epileptiform convulsions
- **C.** depression of uterine activity
- **D.** potentiation of depolarising muscle relaxants
- **E.** potentiation of non-depolarising muscle relaxants

Q 37. Acute herpes zoster infection:

- **A.** typically involves thoracic dermatomes
- **B.** is caused by an RNA virus
- **C.** treated promptly with steroids will not progress to post herpetic neuralgia
- **D.** may cause pain lasting more than 3 months
- **E.** involves first and second order sensory neurones

Q 38. Surgical correction of scoliosis:

- **A.** carries a high risk of spinal cord damage
- **B.** is facilitated by induced hypotension
- **C.** is monitored by somatosensory evoked potentials
- **D.** may involve division of the diaphragm
- **E.** typically requires postoperative ventilation for several days

Q 39. In a 2-week-old term infant with pyloric stenosis and dehydration the appropriate fluids to be given iv are:

A. 5% dextrose with 0.45% saline
B. 8.4% sodium bicarbonate
C. potassium chloride
D. calcium gluconate
E. Ringer's lactate

Q 40. Cerebral blood flow:

A. is controlled by local variations in metabolic activity
B. is controlled by changes in extracellular pH
C. is affected by changes in $PaCO_2$
D. is 25% of cardiac output
E. in healthy individuals is related to systemic blood pressure

Q 41. A 50-year-old man is admitted following an acute myocardial infarction. He developed persistent ST elevation during his stay in hospital. The ST segment change:

A. is probably insignificant
B. can indicate pericarditis
C. will be due to β-blockers
D. is associated with a left ventricular aneurysm
E. is treated with digoxin

Q 42. Features of tension pneumothorax include:

A. raised jugular venous pressure (JVP)
B. pulsus paradoxus
C. tracheal deviation towards the lesion
D. loss of cardiac dullness to percussion
E. Cullen's sign

Q 43. The knee jerk:

A. is due to stretch of tendon reflexes
B. is propagated via S1, S2 and S3 nerve roots
C. involves the femoral nerves
D. is instantly abolished following spinal cord trauma
E. is exaggerated following cervical cord trauma

Paper 1 Questions

Q 44. Premature neonates:

- **A.** are prone to develop hypocalcaemia
- **B.** are sensitive to non-depolarising muscle relaxant drugs
- **C.** have reduced insensible water loss
- **D.** have increased plasma unconjugated bilirubin levels
- **E.** have excess type 1 (oxidative) muscle fibres in the diaphragm

Q 45. In assessing the adequacy of medullary perfusion during posterior fossa surgery the appearance of the following are useful:

- **A.** irregularities in perfusion
- **B.** cardiac arrhythmias
- **C.** hypothermia
- **D.** increase in mean arterial pressure
- **E.** δ waves in the electroencephalogram

Q 46. Tramadol hydrochloride:

- **A.** produces mydriasis
- **B.** has an anti-nociceptive action that is fully blocked by naloxone
- **C.** has a greater affinity for μ-receptors than morphine
- **D.** has a peripheral site of action
- **E.** acts to reduce the synaptic concentration of serotonin and noradrenaline

Q 47. The following are nephrotoxic:

- **A.** aminoglycosides
- **B.** isoflurane
- **C.** non-steroidal anti-inflammatory drugs (NSAIDs)
- **D.** angiotensin converting enzyme inhibitor
- **E.** radiocontrast agents

Q 48. During intermittent positive pressure mechanical ventilation:

- **A.** an increase in peak airway pressure indicates an increase in total lung compliance
- **B.** a rise in plateau pressure indicates a fall in total lung and chest wall compliance

C. a falling peak pressure can indicate a leak in the breathing circuit
D. a pneumothorax will produce an increase in peak and plateau pressures
E. bronchial constriction may be shown by a rise in peak airway pressure

Q 49. Intraoperative signs of a haemolytic transfusion reaction include:

A. hypertension
B. pyrexia
C. urticaria
D. an increase in capillary bleeding
E. periorbital oedema

Q 50. Characteristic features of the myasthenic syndrome include:

A. increase sensitivity to depolarising neuromuscular blocking drugs
B. decreased eletromyogram (EMG) voltage
C. resistance to non-depolarising neuromuscular blocking drugs
D. post tetanic facilitation
E. fade of the EMG

Q 51. Phaeochromocytomas:

A. are noradrenaline secreting tumours
B. can occur anywhere along the sympathetic chain
C. are usually benign
D. produce hypotension
E. produce excessive amounts of adrenaline

Q 52. In haemophilia:

A. purpura is rare
B. the bleeding time is prolonged
C. the coagulation time is prolonged
D. the capillary resistant test is normal
E. the clot retraction is normal

Paper 1 Questions

Q 53. Circulatory changes during the administration of enflurane includes decrease in the:

A. systemic vascular resistance
B. right atrial pressure
C. cerebral blood flow
D. renal blood flow
E. splanchnic blood flow

Q 54. Atropine:

A. blocks the muscarinic effects of acetylcholine
B. given as a premedication is contraindicated in glaucoma
C. crosses the blood brain barrier
D. inhibits acetylcholine release
E. can cause pyrexia

Q 55. The following statements are correct:

A. Main stream capnographs significantly increase dead space
B. Side stream capnographs are suitable for use with nasal cannulae
C. Side stream capnographs under read
D. The response time of side stream capnographs is more rapid than main stream capnographs
E. End-tidal carbon dioxide concentration reflects changes in cardiac output

Q 56. Inaccurate interpretation of left ventricular end-diastolic pressure by pulmonary arterial occlusion wedge pressure measurements occurs in:

A. tricuspid regurgitation
B. aortic regurgitation
C. pulmonary hypertension
D. mitral stenosis
E. mitral incompetence

Q 57. Likely causes of a mixed venous hypoxaemia in a hypothermic patient include:

A. failure to correct the value for body temperature
B. undetected left to right cardiac shunt

C. increased oxygen consumption from shivering
D. increased oxygen dissolved in plasma
E. low cardiac output

Q 58. Diamorphine:

A. is a naturally occurring opioid
B. is more lipid soluble than morphine
C. has a higher affinity than morphine for opioid receptors
D. is well absorbed after subcutaneous administration
E. is converted to mono-acetyl morphine

Q 59. Mivacurium:

A. penetrates the blood-brain barrier
B. is antagonised by magnesium ions
C. blocks autonomic ganglia
D. is a bisquarternary benzylisoquinoline
E. has an active breakdown product

Q 60. The following are true of the ideal intravascular pressure monitoring system:

A. the resonance frequency should be less than 40 Hz
B. the manometer tubing should be compliant
C. the transducer diaphragm should be stiff
D. the damping coefficient is 0.7
E. the manometer tubing should be a small diameter

Q 61. Isoflurane vapour:

A. concentration can be measured using a refractometer
B. is less dense than nitrous oxide
C. will absorb ultraviolet radiation
D. concentration can be measured by absorption of infrared radiation
E. concentration can be measured by the changes in the elasticity of silicon rubber

Q 62. Applications of the Doppler effect in the measurement of blood flow involves changes in:

A. electrical conductivity of a moving stream of blood
B. frequency response on the arterial wall

C. frequency reflected ultrasound waves
D. temperate of blood as it moves peripherally
E. harmonic waves of reflected arterial pulses

Q 63. The air in the operating theatre:

A. has a dew point of 37°C
B. is tested for pollution with anaesthetic gases by means of an infrared analyser
C. is used in the calibration of an oxygen analyser
D. has a higher pO_2 when the temperature is raised
E. contains more oxygen per ml than does arterial blood for a normal subject

Q 64. The treatment of amitriptyline poisoning includes:

A. forced diuresis
B. an isoprenaline infusion
C. digitalisation
D. intravenous atropine sulphate
E. β adrenoceptor antagonists

Q 65. Gas chromatography:

A. utilises the principle of selectively retarding the passage of gases through a tube
B. is used to detect enflurane
C. quantifies the individual components of a mixture of gases
D. uses carbon dioxide as a carrier gas
E. is suitable for measuring nitrous oxide concentrations

Q 66. In cardiac output measurement by thermal dilution:

A. the thermistor is accurate to 1°C
B. measurements under-read cardiac output after 48 h in situ
C. the thermistor measures true core temperature
D. the measurements under-read cardiac output during inspiration
E. the thermistor lead is situated proximal to the balloon

Q 67. A direct indication of scatter in a group of experimental results is provided by:

A. the mean
B. centiles
C. the standard deviation
D. $P < 0.05$
E. the square of the standard error

Q 68. Characteristic findings in acute respiratory failure associated with chronic bronchitis include:

A. a raised jugular venous pressure
B. muscular twitching
C. papilloedema
D. a small volume pulse
E. cold extremities

Q 69. Pulmonary hypertension is a complication of:

A. atrial septal defect
B. ventricular septal defect
C. patent ductus arteriosus
D. pulmonary embolism
E. sodium nitroprusside therapy

Q 70. The treatment of acute complete heart block includes:

A. iv glucagon
B. transvenous pacing
C. iv isoprenaline
D. atropine
E. digoxin

Q 71. The carotid sheath contains the:

A. common carotid artery
B. internal jugular vein
C. sympathetic trunk
D. vagus nerve
E. phrenic nerve

Q 72. **Convulsions occur with:**

A. penicillin
B. tetracycline
C. phenobarbitone
D. acetazolomide
E. frusemide

Q 73. **When regional anaesthesia is compared to general anaesthesia for hip fractures it is associated with:**

A. reduced post-operative mortality
B. reduced blood loss
C. reduce risk of DVT
D. reduced hospital stay
E. better immediate postoperative pain relief

Q 74. **Rate of diffusion of a gas is:**

A. proportional to the thickness of the membrane
B. directly proportional to the tension gradient
C. inversely proportional to the square root of the molecular weight
D. increased as the temperature of the liquid decreases
E. does not depend on the ambient pressure

Q 75. **The prothrombin time is prolonged in:**

A. heparin therapy
B. von Willebrand's disease
C. scurvy
D. thrombocytopenia
E. jaundice

Q 76. **In Fallot's tetralogy there is:**

A. splitting of the first heart sound
B. a murmur caused by blood flowing through a ventricular septal defect
C. squatting
D. syncope
E. oligaemic lung fields

Q 77. Suxamethonium is contraindicated in:

A. dystrophia myotonica
B. neonates
C. congestive heart failure
D. acute intermittent porphyria
E. Parkinson's disease

Q 78. The immediate management of hyperthermia due to severe exercise includes:

A. immediate cooling
B. aspirin
C. sodium bicarbonate
D. chlorpromazine
E. iv crystalloid

Q 79. The addition of continuous positive airway pressure (CPAP) into the breathing system causes a reduction in the:

A. FRC
B. static compliance of the lung
C. dynamic compliance of the lung
D. airway conductance
E. work of breathing

Q 80. Decompression sickness:

A. is associated with a vascular necrosis of bone
B. is due to an alveolar oxygen deficit
C. is cured by breathing in a mixture of oxygen and helium
D. can occur four hours after the initial drop in pressure
E. is avoided if nitrogen is included in the inspired gas mixture

Q 81. Patients in diabetic coma can have:

A. lactic acidosis
B. hyperosmolarity
C. ketoacidosis
D. hyperlipidaemia
E. hypocalcaemia

Q 82. The following drugs counteract the effect of isoprenaline on the heart:

A. propranolol
B. atropine
C. diazoxide
D. trimetaphan
E. nifedipine

Q 83. Loss of ankle reflexes is associated with:

A. multiple sclerosis
B. taboparesis
C. ataxia
D. bulbar palsy
E. subacute combined degeneration of the cord

Q 84. If effective α-adrenergic blockade were achieved in a patient one would expect:

A. hypotension
B. orthostatic hypotension
C. miosis
D. cold pale skin
E. bradycardia

Q 85. The following can occur after dextran infusion:

A. decreased coagulability
B. difficulties with cross matching of blood
C. renal tubular damage
D. rouleaux formation
E. an antigenic reaction

Q 86. Aortic stenosis may be caused by:

A. congenital malformation
B. rheumatic fever
C. subacute bacterial endocarditis (SBE)
D. calcified aortic cusps
E. ruptured aortic cusps

Q 87. The following are effective in attenuating the pressor response to intubation:

A. intravenous lidocaine
B. calcium antagonists
C. angiotensin-converting enzyme (ACE) inhibitors
D a large dose of an induction agent
E. β-blockers

Q 88. An elevated left hemidiaphragm can be caused by:

A. left phrenic nerve paralysis
B. left lower lobe collapse
C. sinus inversus
D. left pleural effusion
E. left pneumothorax

Q 89. The following increase the risk of cauda equina syndrome (CES):

A. old age
B. the use of epidural adrenaline
C. the lithotomy position
D. the use of barbotage
E. the prone position

Q 90. DC cardio-version is indicated for:

A. supraventricular tachycardia
B. ventricular tachycardia
C. premature atrial contraction
D. digitalis toxicity
E. premature ventricular contraction

Table for your Answers

Question	A	B	C	D	E
1					
2					
3					
4					
5					
6					
7					
8					
9					
10					
11					
12					
13					
14					
15					
16					
17					
18					
19					
20					
21					
22					
23					
24					
25					
26					
27					
28					
29					
30					

Question	A	B	C	D	E
31					
32					
33					
34					
35					
36					
37					
38					
39					
40					
41					
42					
43					
44					
45					
46					
47					
48					
49					
50					
51					
52					
53					
54					
55					
56					
57					
58					
59					
60					

Question	A	B	C	D	E
61					
62					
63					
64					
65					
66					
67					
68					
69					
70					
71					
72					
73					
74					
75					
76					
77					
78					
79					
80					
81					
82					
83					
84					
85					
86					
87					
88					
89					
90					

Paper 2 Questions

Q 1. An asthmatic patient develops acute bronchospasm at the end of an operation for the repair of an umbilical hernia. The possible causes include:

A. use of neostigmine to reverse the neuromuscular blockade
B. a light level of anaesthesia
C. irritation of the respiratory tree by the tracheal tube
D. use of isoflurane during the anaesthetic
E. inclusion of morphine in the preoperative medication

Q 2. During anaesthesia a patient with Parkinson's disease taking levodopa should not receive:

A. enflurane
B. fentanyl
C. morphine
D. droperidol
E. nitrous oxide

Q 3. After the onset of one lung anaesthesia pulmonary vasoconstriction in the non-dependant lung is enhanced by:

A. a low alveolar oxygen tension in that lung
B. inhalational anaesthetic agents
C. intravenous anaesthetic agents
D. metabolic alkalosis
E. a constant intravenous sodium nitroprusside infusion

Q 4. Reliable indicators of tissue oxygenation include the following:

A. base deficit in arterial blood
B. pH of arterial blood
C. PO_2 of arterial blood

Paper 2 Questions

D. pH of venous blood
E. PO_2 of venous blood

Q 5. Pancreatitis is associated with:

A. respiratory distress syndrome
B. hypercalcaemia
C. alcoholism
D. cholelithiasis
E. polyarteritis nodosa

Q 6. Subarachnoid haemorrhage:

A. is precipitated by dehydration
B. can be detected on a CT scan
C. is more common in males
D. causes an increase in intracranial pressure
E. is associated with a maximal incidence of vasospasm from the third to the tenth day after the bleed

Q 7. Characteristic features of myotonia congenita include:

A. amenorrhoea
B. involvement of the long flexors of the hands
C. fasciculations in the affected muscles
D. worsening on exposure to heat
E. improvement after repeated voluntary activity

Q 8. Lower oesophageal sphincter tone is increased by:

A. metoclopramide
B. domperidone
C. cisapride
D. atropine
E. morphine

Q 9. Postoperative nausea and vomiting (PONV):

A. is commoner in men than in women
B. is more common over 70 years old compared to those under 50 years old
C. is prevented by the action of 5-HT_3 agonists in the brain

D. is stimulated by vagal afferents
E. can be dangerous in ocular surgery

Q 10. In critically ill patients the direct pharmacokinetics of a drug are affected by:

A. tissue oedema
B. hypoxia
C. respiratory acidaemia
D. receptor upregulation
E. central nervous system dysfunction

Q 11. The following groups of people have an increased risk of latex allergy:

A. healthcare workers
B. those who have had repeated tracheal intubation
C. those who have had repeated surgical procedures
D. those with an allergy to fruit
E. those with penicillin allergy

Q 12. Angiotensin-converting enzyme (ACE) inhibitors:

A. increase total body water
B. cause a cough
C. cause peripheral vasodilatation
D. cause a bradycardia
E. decrease the pressor response to laryngoscopy

Q 13. Haemoptysis is seen in:

A. mitral stenosis
B. pulmonary infarction
C. bronchiectasis
D. Mallory Weiss syndrome
E. Good Pasteur's syndrome

Q 14. Deep cervical plexus block can cause:

A. bradycardia
B. dyspnoea
C. Bell's palsy

D. mydriasis
E. hoarseness of the voice

Q 15. Lateral popliteal nerve block (common peroneal nerve) can cause loss of:

A. dorsiflexion of the great toe
B. sensation between the hallux and the second toe
C. evasion of the foot
D. plantar flexion of the foot
E. ankle jerk

Q 16. The treatment of anaphylaxis includes:

A. 0.1 mg/kg of 1:1,000 im adrenaline
B. 1 mg/kg of 1:10,000 iv adrenaline
C. intravenous steroids
D. nebulised adrenaline
E. a maximum dose of adrenaline of 1 mg for an adult

Q 17. The appropriate management of stridor in infants following cleft palate surgery includes:

A. nebulised adrenaline
B. surgical tracheostomy
C. humidified oxygen
D. intravenous hydrocortisone
E. tracheal intubation

Q 18. With regards to surgery on the third and fourth toes without the use of a tourniquet the following nerves should be blocked:

A. deep peroneal nerve
B. common peroneal nerve
C. saphenous nerve
D. tibial nerve
E. sural nerve

Q 19. Chronic myeloid leukaemia is associated with:

A. genetic translocation
B. frequent bone fractures

C. massive splenomegaly
D. a platelet count less than in chronic lymphatic leukaemia
E. lower limb paralysis

Q 20. In patients with long standing Cushing's disease, the following are associated with a high incidence of perioperative complications:

A. hypokalaemia
B. muscle wasting
C. hypernatraemia
D. hypertension
E. diabetes mellitus

Q 21. Obstructive sleep apnoea:

A. occurs in about 1% of the general population
B. can be treated by nasal continuous positive airway pressure (CPAP)
C. is caused by pharyngeal obstruction rather than obstruction caused by the tongue
D. can be caused by central factors rather than abnormal anatomy
E. can present with right heart failure

Q 22. Transmission of hepatitis B virus can occur with:

A. plasma
B. fibrinogen
C. packed red cells
D. albumin
E. platelet concentrates

Q 23. Neuropraxia:

A. is more common after long operations than short operations
B. does not occur with local anaesthetics
C. does not occur with the use of muscle relaxants
D. only occurs when pre-existing neuropathy is present
E. characteristically takes 6 to 12 months to recover

Q 24. During oxygen therapy, pulmonary oxygen toxicity is more likely to be associated with:

A. increased CO_2 tensions
B. increased duration of exposure
C. high altitude
D. anaemia
E. increased muscular activity

Q 25. In a patient with sickle cell anaemia:

A. epidural analgesia is contraindicated
B. the haemoglobin concentration should be restored to normal levels prior to surgery
C. plasma expanders are contraindicated
D. bone pain heralds a sickle cell crisis
E. preparation should be made for exchange transfusion of the neonate following delivery to a homozygous mother

Q 26. Ankylosing spondylitis:

A. occurs more frequently in women than men over the age of 40
B. is associated with low grade pyrexia
C. can present as sciatica
D. can be complicated by arthropathy affecting the hips
E. can be complicated by iritis

Q 27. Causes of right bundle branch block include:

A. atrial septal defect
B. myxoedema
C. myocardial ischaemia
D. pulmonary embolism
E. myotonia congenita

Q 28. Blood flow within the brain is:

A. altered locally by changes in the cerebral vascular resistance
B. increased in the area adjacent to a tumour
C. affected by alterations in extracellular pH
D. primarily dependent on systemic arterial pressure
E. reduced in REM sleep

Q 29. When spontaneous ventilation is first instituted after a patient has had 24 h of passive hyperventilation the:

- **A.** arterial blood pH is greater than normal
- **B.** $PaCO_2$ is lower than normal
- **C.** carbon dioxide response curve is shifted to the left
- **D.** concentration of bicarbonate in cerebrospinal fluid is decreased
- **E.** P50 is greater than before hyperventilation

Q 30. In the measurement of arterial blood pressure using a transducer:

- **A.** the catheter should be long and narrow
- **B.** the catheter should be stiff walled
- **C.** an 18 G cannula is most appropriate
- **D.** systolic pressure in the aortic arch normally exceeds left ventricular end-systolic pressure
- **E.** systolic pressure in the dorsalis pedis artery normally exceeds the radial artery pressure

Q 31. The thermistor bead:

- **A.** can be used in the measurement of blood flow
- **B.** has a very large thermal capacity
- **C.** can measure very small temperature changes
- **D.** has a linear response to resistance change with temperature
- **E.** responds more quickly to temperature change than a mercury in glass thermometer

Q 32. The following occur in Cushing's syndrome:

- **A.** proximal myopathy
- **B.** generalised obesity
- **C.** psychosis
- **D.** sodium retention
- **E.** glucosuria

Q 33. The following are true about the foetal circulation:

- **A.** the PO_2 in the descending aorta is lower than that in the aortic arch
- **B.** the ductus venosus contains mixed venous blood

C. the ductus arteriosus closes due to the rise in the systemic pressure
D. closure of the foramen ovale is due to the change in left and right atrial pressures
E. blood from the inferior vena cava can reach the systemic circulation without passing through the left side of the heart

Q 34. Constant pulse rate after a Valsalva manoeuvre may occur in:

A. Horner's syndrome
B. uncomplicated aortic regurgitation
C. diabetes mellitus
D. malignant hypertension
E. autonomic neuropathy

Q 35. The following conditions are associated with difficult intubation:

A. Marfan's syndrome
B. Acromegaly
C. Charcot-Marie Tooth syndrome
D. Ludwig's angina
E. Down's syndrome

Q 36. A negative nitrogen balance is to be expected:

A. during pregnancy
B. in acute renal failure
C. postoperatively
D. in acute ulcerative colitis
E. during steroid administration

Q 37. The following are recognised causes of thrombocytopenia:

A. cirrhosis of the liver
B. treatment with thiazide diuretics
C. splenectomy
D. systemic lupus erythematosus
E. infectious mononucleosis

Q 38. In patients suffering from major trauma, hyperkalaemia may result from:

A. dopamine therapy
B. hyperventilation
C. lactic acidosis
D. acute renal failure
E. rhabdomyolysis

Q 39. Fluoroquinolones are:

A. a cause of fits
B. chelated by aluminium salts
C. chemically related to nalidixic acid
D. effective against pneumococci
E. effective in gram negative pneumonia

Q 40. Rapid shallow breathing in critically ill patients:

A. is seen in acute respiratory failure
B. is associated with failure to wean from a ventilator
C. is due to respiratory muscle weakness
D. is due to hypoxaemia
E. results from a high $PaCO_2$

Q 41. Appropriate ventilator adjustments in a patient with a flail chest, in whom air is escaping from the chest drain at a rate of 1.5 l/min include:

A. increasing the inspiratory flow rate
B. decreasing the respiratory rate
C. subtracting 1.5 l from the desired minute ventilation
D. adding 10 cm positive end expiratory pressure (PEEP)
E. decreasing peak inspiratory pressure

Q 42. Pulmonary vascular resistance is:

A. increased if the haemocrit is abnormally high
B. increased by the application of 5 cmH_2O PEEP
C. decreased when breathing 79% helium in 21% oxygen
D. increased by breathing 2% sevoflurane in air
E. decreased by moderate exercise

Paper 2

Questions

Q 43. In normal pregnancy:

- **A.** the plasma colloid osmotic pressure decreases to about 17 mmHg
- **B.** the total quantity of plasma proteins is decreased
- **C.** the concentration of most globulins increases
- **D.** plasma volume increases to 60 ml/kg
- **E.** altered plasma protein levels increase the toxicity of local anaesthetic agents

Q 44. After a successful supraclavicular brachial plexus block, sensory anaesthesia will usually be incomplete on the:

- **A.** medial aspect of the forearm
- **B.** lateral aspect of the forearm
- **C.** lateral aspect of the upper arm
- **D.** medial aspect of the arm
- **E.** back of elbow

Q 45. When a mismatched blood transfusion occurs in an anaesthetised patient, early findings include:

- **A.** oozing
- **B.** hypertension
- **C.** respiratory arrest
- **D.** tachypnoea
- **E.** tachycardia

Q 46. Regarding nitric oxide:

- **A.** it is a neurotransmitter
- **B.** it has a half-life of 8 min
- **C.** inducible nitric oxide synthase is Ca^{2+} dependant
- **D.** excessive administration leads to the formation of methaemoglobin
- **E.** more than 15 ppm is required for the treatment of acute respiratory distress syndrome (ARDS)

Q 47. The characteristic features of small bowel obstruction include:

- **A.** nausea and vomiting
- **B.** absent bowel sounds

C. percussion dullness in the flanks
D. absolute constipation
E. constant pains whatever the position

Q 48. Mixed venous oxygen saturation is reduced in:

A. anaemia
B. hypothermia
C. sepsis
D. shivering
E. low cardiac output

Q 49. Base deficit:

A. only measures the pH of plasma
B. is the amount of acid or base to be added to plasma to bring the pH of blood to 7.4
C. can be used to assess respiratory acidosis
D. is a measure of the metabolic component of an acid base disorder
E. is affected by doubling or halving the (H^+), which will change the pH by $\log_{10}(0.3)$

Q 50. The following drugs are safe to be used in patients with malignant hyperthermia:

A. nitrous oxide
B. fentanyl
C. propofol
D. droperidol
E. atropine

Q 51. With regard to laser surgery:

A. the Sander's injector can be used on the side of the bronchoscope
B. the patient's eyes are not at risk
C. the wearing of goggles is not necessary for staff working 1 m from the surgical field
D. aluminium foil is used to wrap the tracheal tube
E. laser equipment is categorised as Class III medical equipment

Paper 2 Questions

Q 52. The following agents can be used as an anticoagulant during continuous veno-venous haemofiltration:

A. warfarin
B. aspirin
C. PGE1
D. heparin
E. low molecular heparin

Q 53. Phenytoin:

A. is the treatment of choice in status epilepticus
B. loading dose is 7 mg/kg iv
C. can be given via a peripheral line
D. dose can be increased beyond the therapeutic level to achieve a desirable response
E. has membrane stabilising activity

Q 54. Idiopathic infantile respiratory distress syndrome:

A. is common after 36 weeks of gestation
B. usually occurs after caesarean section
C. usually occurs within 12 h of delivery
D. is treated with iv steroids
E. is more common in multiple pregnancies

Q 55. The immediate complications following partial thyroidectomy include:

A. stridor
B. thyroid crisis
C. hypocalcaemia
D. respiratory obstruction
E. myxoedema

Q 56. Concerning bilirubin metabolism:

A. there is increased conjugated bilirubin with extra hepatic obstruction
B. there is increased unconjugated bilirubin with haemolysis
C. unconjugated bilirubin causes cerebral damage in neonates
D. a patient previously treated with phenobarbitone will have increased bilirubin formation
E. bilirubin diglucuronide formation takes place in the liver

Q 57. **Hypofibrinogenaemia is associated with:**

A. amniotic fluid embolism
B. incompatible blood transfusion
C. septic abortion
D. prostate resection
E. patients receiving oral contraceptive therapy

Q 58. **Xenon:**

A. has an anaesthetic property at ambient pressure
B. supports combustion
C. contains free fluoride atoms
D. is present in air at concentrations of 0.2%
E. is converted to inactive metabolites by hepatic microsomes

Q 59. **The emergency management of severe head injury includes:**

A. the maintenance of normotension
B. the avoidance of hyperglycaemia
C. hyperventilation to $PaCO_2$ of 3.5 kPa
D. the early administration of mannitol 10 g per kg
E. reducing $CMRO_2$ with high doses of thiopentone

Q 60. **The treatment of chest pain in a patient who has a heart rate of 100/min and BP 140/90 and suffers from aortic stenosis includes:**

A. supplemental oxygen
B. diazepam
C. esmolol
D. sublingual GTN
E. sodium nitroprusside

Q 61. **The following can measure oxygen in a mixture of gases:**

A. pulmonary oximeter
B. infrared analyser
C. flame photodetector
D. Van Slyke apparatus
E. mass spectrometer

Paper 2 Questions

Q 62. Post operative delayed recovery 45 min following induction of anaesthesia with 100 mg suxamethonium can be due to:

A. phase 2 desensitisation
B. acetylcholine block
C. pseudocholine esterase deficiency
D. concurrent administration of opioids
E. subclinical renal impairment

Q 63. The following are associated with portal hypertension:

A. haemochromocytosis
B. Budd Chiari syndrome
C. Wilson's disease
D. Gilbert's disease
E. oral contraceptive therapy

Q 64. Humidity can be measured by:

A. mass spectrometry
B. chromatography
C. the dew point
D. biological organ length
E. weight

Q 65. Rheumatoid arthritis is associated with:

A. aortic stenosis
B. tricuspid regurgitation
C. symmetrical arthropathy
D. acanthosis nigricans
E. mononeuritis multiplex

Q 66. Peribulbar block:

A. avoids intraorbital haematomas
B. is not suitable for prolonged procedures
C. local anaesthetic is deposited between the inferior and lateral rectus muscles
D. can cause eyeball injury in myopic eyes with an axial length of more than 25 mm
E. the needle never goes beyond 3 cm depth

Q 67. Complex regional pain syndrome is characterised by:

A. a reduction in skin temperature
B. pain in the affected limb
C. aleukocytosis
D. an increased incidence in athletes
E. eventual development of osteoporosis

Q 68. The following are risk factors for postoperative nausea and vomiting:

A. a history of motion sickness
B. propofol anaesthesia
C. nitrous oxide
D. middle ear surgery
E. female gender

Q 69. In patients with renal failure, the following drugs or their active metabolites may accumulate if given repeatedly:

A. thiopentone
B. propofol
C. vecuronium
D. morphine
E. erythromycin

Q 70. A three-year old boy with pallor and bruising has anaemia, thrombocytopenia and a low white cell count with occasional blast cells. The likely diagnosis includes:

A. idiopathic thrombocytopenia
B. a leukaemic reaction
C. chronic lymphatic leukaemia
D. myelosclerosis
E. acute leukaemia

Q 71. Collapse of the right lower lobe of the lung is characterised by:

A. tachypnoea
B. an increased alveolar to arterial oxygen tension difference
C. an increased $PaCO_2$
D. an area of stony dullness to percussion
E. a decreased pH of arterial blood

Q 72. The alveolar arterial oxygen tension difference is increased by:

A. nitrous oxide uptake
B. a high inspired oxygen concentration
C. a reduction in FRC
D. hepatic failure
E. increase in ventilation/perfusion mismatch

Q 73. PEEP increases:

A. residual volume
B. functional residual capacity
C. expiratory residual volume
D. closing volume
E. total lung capacity

Q 74. The following are found in venous blood. Na^+ 127 mmol/l, K^+ 6.2 mmol/l, Cl^- 85 mmol/l, HCO_3^- 19 mmol/l. These results suggest:

A. renal failure
B. hepatic failure
C. adrenal cortical insufficiency
D. high bowel obstruction with vomiting
E. diabetes insipidus

Q 75. When assessing neuromuscular blockade:

A. supra-maximal stimulation is achieved only when the voltage is turned to maximum
B. supra-maximal stimulation is used only when there is more than 75% block
C. supra-maximal stimulation is used only when tetanus is applied
D. no response to stimulation always indicates 100% block
E. post-tetanic facilitation means that a twitch after a tetanus is larger than the tetanus

Q 76. In children death due to severe burns on the second week after injury is often due to:

A. anaemia
B. hepatic failure

C. haemoconcentration
D. toxaemia from protein destruction
E. infection of the burned area

Q 77. The α-2 adrenoceptor agonist clonidine:

A. increases heart rate
B. reduces arterial blood pressure
C. reduces the dose requirement for inhalational anaesthetics
D. increases the duration of epidurally administered bupivacaine
E. antagonises the analgesic effect of opioids

Q 78. Lactic acid is:

A. formed during anaerobic ATP re-synthesis
B. not formed by red blood cells
C. increased in concentration in the blood during energy deficit
D. converted to glucose by the Cori cycle
E. oxidised without conversion back to glucose

Q 79. Dopamine:

A. demonstrates a renal protective reflex
B. increases creatinine clearance
C. increases intracellular calcium concentration
D. usually increases cardiac output at 2 μg/kg/min
E. increases splanchnic oxygen requirement

Q 80. During the first stage of labour:

A. umbilical arterial PCO_2 is 7 kPa
B. umbilical arterial PO_2 is 7 kPa
C. umbilical venous PCO_2 is 5.5 kPa
D. uterine artery PCO_2 is 5 kPa
E. uterine arterial PO_2 is 12.5 kPa

Q 81. The treatment of ventricular tachycardia under anaesthesia includes:

A. lidocaine (lignocaine)
B. amiodarone

C. rapid digitalisation
D. propranolol
E. DC shock

Q 82. The pain of chronic pancreatitis can be relieved by:

A. thoracic epidural block
B. coeliac plexus block
C. paravertebral block
D. lumbar sympathetic block
E. intrathecal phenol

Q 83. Phantom limb pain is:

A. more common if there was pain in the limb before the amputation
B. treated with anticonvulsant
C. can be precipitated by performing a spinal block
D. treated by sympathetic blockade
E. not a feature of traumatic limb amputation

Q 84. The level of spinal block is dependent on the:

A. baracity of local anaesthetics
B. position of the patient
C. volume of CSF
D. volume of local anaesthetics
E. concentration of local anaesthetics

Q 85. Inhalational induction in children with sevoflurane is faster because of their:

A. increased minimum alveolar concentration (MAC)
B. increased cardiac output per kg compared to adults
C. increased minute ventilation per kg compared to adults
D. increased tissue solubility
E. small FRC

Q 86. Enteral nutrition:

A. cannot be used in the absence of bowel sounds
B. prevents the overgrowth of gut pathogens

C. is contraindicated 4 h post-abdominal surgery
D. post pyloric catheter feed is becoming the more popular route
E. reduces the incidence of calculus cholecystitis

Q 87. The hazards of diathermy in the operating theatre can be minimised by:

A. the use of needle electrodes
B. placing the patient's plate as close to the surgical site as possible
C. the use of a capacitor between the patient and the diathermy
D. avoidance of battery powered equipment
E. the use of inductance

Q 88. Spinal anaesthesia with the block level at T2 is associated with:

A. hypertension
B. mydriasis
C. tachycardia
D. ventricular extrasystoles
E. nodal rhythm

Q 89. With regard to dental chair anaesthesia the following are contraindications:

A. sickle cell anaemia
B. angina
C. dental abscess
D. learning difficulties
E. Down's syndrome

Q 90. Postoperative respiratory micro-atelectasis is associated with:

A. decreased $PaCO_2$
B. scattered areas of dullness on percussion over the chest
C. ground glass appearances on chest X-ray
D. use of opioids intra-operatively
E. bilateral basal crepitations on auscultation

Table for your Answers

Paper 2 Questions

Question	A	B	C	D	E
1					
2					
3					
4					
5					
6					
7					
8					
9					
10					
11					
12					
13					
14					
15					
16					
17					
18					
19					
20					
21					
22					
23					
24					
25					
26					
27					
28					
29					
30					

Question	A	B	C	D	E
31					
32					
33					
34					
35					
36					
37					
38					
39					
40					
41					
42					
43					
44					
45					
46					
47					
48					
49					
50					
51					
52					
53					
54					
55					
56					
57					
58					
59					
60					

Paper 2

Questions

Question	A	B	C	D	E
61					
62					
63					
64					
65					
66					
67					
68					
69					
70					
71					
72					
73					
74					
75					
76					
77					
78					
79					
80					
81					
82					
83					
84					
85					
86					
87					
88					
89					
90					

Paper 3 Questions

Q 1. Changes in pulmonary function and lung volume occurring during pregnancy include:

A. decreased functional residual capacity (FRC)
B. decreased total lung capacity
C. increased expiratory reserve volume
D. decreased airway conductance (increased airway pressure)
E. decreased $PaCO_2$

Q 2. The hazards of anaesthesia in a patient with chronic renal failure include:

A. left ventricular enlargement
B. cardiac tamponade
C. hypertension
D. pericarditis
E. enhanced carotid sinus activity

Q 3. Trans-oesophageal echocardiography:

A. is helpful in assessing myocardial contractility
B. is helpful is assessing myocardial ischaemic
C. can give an index of stroke volume
D. is useful for observing tricuspid regurgitation
E. can be used to measure intraventricular pressure changes

Q 4. Blood gas results showing PaO_2 8 kPa, $PaCO_2$ 4 kPa, pH 7.4 are consistent with:

A. compensated metabolic alkalosis
B. alveolar hypoventilation
C. pulmonary atelectasis
D. acute coronary occlusion
E. residence at high altitude for 48 h

Q 5. The postoperative anabolic phase is characterised by:

A. the mobilisation of body fat
B. nitrogen anabolism at the rate of 3 to 5 g/day
C. a requirement ideally for a calorie nitrogen intake of 150 calories per gram of nitrogen
D. an increase in the excretion of potassium
E. the synthesis of 30 g lean wet muscle tissue per gram of nitrogen retained

Q 6. Lipid solubility of inhalational anaesthetic agents affects:

A. potency
B. speed of induction
C. volatility
D. recovery
E. compatibility with soda-lime

Q 7. Conditions associated with smoke inhalational injury include:

A. sloughing of the mucosa of the upper airway
B. the immediate development of pulmonary oedema
C. a shift of the oxygen dissociation curve to the left
D. heat injury to the lung parenchyma
E. increased carboxyhaemoglobin concentration

Q 8. In a patient with chronic obstructive airway disease and an elevated $PaCO_2$:

A. hypoxic respiratory drive is likely to be important
B. bicarbonate infusion will increase the $PaCO_2$
C. pH is usually less than 7.25
D. arterial oxygen saturation is less than 75%
E. serum bicarbonate is elevated

Q 9. In non-invasive blood pressure measurement:

A. the cuff width should be 20% greater than the arm diameter
B. a too narrow cuff will tend to under read blood pressure
C. there are five Korotkoff sounds
D. Doppler frequency shift occurs with blood flow

E. an automated monitor detects pulsations within the cuff as it deflates to systolic pressure, which increases in amplitude until mean arterial blood pressure is reached

Q 10. Sickle cell trait:

A. is found in patients homozygous for HBS
B. causes severe anaemia
C. is associated with reduced P50
D. can be differentiated from sickle cell disease on electrophoresis
E. causes haemolysis

Q 11. Coarctation of the aorta:

A. is usually preductal
B. surgical correction is via a right thoracotomy
C. can be diagnosed on chest X-ray
D. is associated with Berry aneurysms
E. is associated with differential cyanosis

Q 12. The ECG changes produced by alterations in potassium concentration include:

A. long PR interval
B. inverted U waves
C. tented T waves
D. J waves
E. δ waves

Q 13. In acute tubular necrosis:

A. there is initially a small volume of concentrated urine
B. there is malignant hypertension
C. the urea is high and the creatinine is low
D. hyperkalaemia occurs
E. recovery is uncommon

Q 14. Clinical trials:

A. are single blind when only the subject is unaware of the treatment used
B. are double blind when neither the investigator nor the subjects are aware of the treatment given

C. double blind are unsuitable for sequential analysis
D. single blind do not require placebo controls
E. double blind do not prevent observe bias

Q 15. A poorly controlled, insulin dependent diabetic, pregnant mother will have:

A. an increased risk of eclampsia
B. hypoglycaemic episodes in the first trimester
C. a large baby due to the effects of maternal insulin
D. a foetus suffering from chronic hypoxia
E. a foetus with surfactant production proportional to the serum insulin levels

Q 16. The following prevent the re-uptake of noradrenaline:

A. isoprenaline
B. dopamine
C. clomipramine
D. propranolol
E. atropine

Q 17. The passage of local anaesthetics across the placenta depends on the:

A. concentration gradient from maternal to foetal circulation
B. protein binding
C. lipid solubility
D. molecular size
E. water solubility of the hydrophilic acid

Q 18. The following factors do not affect the values obtained from a pulmonary artery flotation catheter:

A. patient temperature
B. injectate temperature
C. site of proximal lumen
D. presence of myocarditis
E. length of time in situ

Q 19. Epistaxis:

A. usually occurs from the lateral wall of the nostril
B. may arise from Small's area

C. may be associated with hypertension
D. may cause anaemia
E. can be relieved by ligation of the ipsilateral vertebral artery in extremis

Q 20. Neurofibromatosis is associated with:

A. pulmonary fibrosis
B. phaeochromocytoma
C. aortic stenosis
D. scoliosis
E. paraplegia

Q 21. In sepsis, flow in the microcirculation is:

A. more homogeneous than in normal individuals
B. regulated by red cell shear stress
C. monitored best by pulmonary artery flotation catheterisation
D. alerted following white cell adhesion molecular expression
E. alerted as a result of increased capillary permeability

Q 22. Oxygen concentrators:

A. contain aluminium silicate
B. produce at least 92% oxygen
C. cannot be used in aircraft
D. can be used to supply a hospital with oxygen
E. provide gas with a concentration of argon, lower than in air

Q 23. The following are powerful paramagnetic gases:

A. oxygen
B. carbon dioxide
C. nitrous oxide
D. nitric oxide
E. halothane

Q 24. In a case of porphyria:

A. griseofulvin may precipitate an acute attack
B. glycine should not be used during transurethral resection of the prostate (TURP)
C. dysautonomia may occur
D. preoperative fluid restriction is beneficial
E. fentanyl can be safely used

Q 25. In mitral stenosis:

- **A.** there is left ventricular hypertrophy
- **B.** the opening snap is secondary to calcified cusps
- **C.** the intensity of the murmur is more significant than its duration
- **D.** systemic anticoagulation is contraindicated for surgery
- **E.** there is a sharp rising carotid upstroke

Q 26. Sevoflurane:

- **A.** has a boiling point of 50.2°C
- **B.** has a blood gas partition coefficient of 0.46
- **C.** contains chloride
- **D.** is degraded into fluoride ions in the body
- **E.** decomposes on exposure to light

Q 27. Important features to prevent hospital-acquired infections in the intensive care unit include:

- **A.** changing the ventilator tubing every 24 h
- **B.** plastic overshoes
- **C.** routine culture of the environment and the equipment
- **D.** separation of new admissions from the rest of the intensive care patients
- **E.** adequate space between the beds as specified in the hospital building standards

Q 28. Trigeminal neuralgia:

- **A.** is associated with absence of the eyelash reflex
- **B.** is successfully treated with gabapentine
- **C.** gasserian block with glycerol is therapeutic
- **D.** is approached through the foramen spinosum
- **E.** is a presenting feature in multiple sclerosis

Q 29. Malignant hyperthermia:

- **A.** is inherited as an autosomal recessive
- **B.** may be precipitated by stress
- **C.** is associated with Duchenne muscular dystrophy
- **D.** is more frequent in males
- **E.** has an incidence of approximately 1 in 15,000 children

Q 30. **The transurethral resection of the prostate (TURP) syndrome:**

A. is associated with hypokalaemia
B. presents with convulsions
C. is prevented by spinal anaesthesia
D. is due to blood loss
E. requires a diuretic for the treatment

Q 31. **The penicillins:**

A. are bactericidal
B. interfere with bacterial cell wall synthesis
C. are more active against organisms, which are not dividing
D. do not affect gram positive cocci
E. are all destroyed by penicillinase

Q 32. **In normal individuals with a normal $PaCO_2$, the cerebral blood flow:**

A. autoregulates between cerebral perfusion pressures of 50 to 100 mmHg
B. is reduced when breathing 100% oxygen
C. increases with hypothermia
D. is normally 45 ml/100 g/min
E. increases following the administration of mannitol

Q 33. **Intercostal nerves:**

A. pass anterior to the posterior intercostal membrane
B. pass between the external and internal intercostal muscles
C. lie superior to the intercostal artery and vein
D. give rise to lateral and anterior cutaneous branches
E. supply the periphery of the diaphragm

Q 34. **Pressure readings obtained, using a pulmonary flotation catheter, in a 50-year-old man were: right atrium 5 mmHg, right ventricle 80/10 mmHg, pulmonary artery 80/60 mmHg, pulmonary wedge 8 mmHg. He could be suffering from:**

A. aortic stenosis
B. mitral stenosis

C. pulmonary hypertension
D. primary myocardial disease
E. ventricular septal defect

Q 35. A patient has the following results: sodium 127 mmol/l, and potassium 6.7 mmol/l. These could be caused by:

A. oliguric renal failure
B. pituitary insufficiency
C. Addison's disease
D. hyperaldosteronism
E. Cushing's syndrome

Q 36. The risk of infection in a central venous catheter:

A. is greater with the internal jugular than with the subclavian approach
B. is greater with the triple lumen than the single lumen catheters
C. depends on the catheter materials
D. is minimised by the use of an occlusive transparent plastic dressing
E. is minimised by the use of a cut down surgical technique

Q 37. In a 5-year-old girl the following suggest a diagnosis of epiglottis rather than croup (acute laryngotracheobronchitis):

A. rapid onset
B. an axillary temperature of 39°C
C. toxaemia (*Haemophilus influenzae* type B)
D. a sore throat
E. a barking cough

Q 38. The hepatic portal vein:

A. has no valves
B. is about 8 cm long
C. is formed from the splenic and the superior mesenteric veins
D. is the main source of oxygen to the liver
E. when obstructed it may cause ascites in the absence of cirrhosis

Q 39. Initial ventilator settings, which would be appropriate in an adult patient with severe acute asthma, include:

A. F_IO_2 of 0.5
B. rate of 15 bpm
C. long inspiratory time
D. peak inspiratory flow rate of 150 l/min
E. PEEP of 10 cmH_2O

Q 40. The following measurements are consistent with physiological oliguria:

A. urine sodium <10 mmol/l
B. urine specific gravity >1.024
C. urine/plasma osmolality ratio 5:1
D. urine/plasma urea ratio 100:1
E. urine/plasma creatinine ratio 20:1

Q 41. Radiological evidence of enlargement of the pulmonary artery is a recognised feature of:

A. atrial septal defect
B. persistent ductus arteriosus
C. mitral stenosis
D. Fallot's tetralogy
E. Eisenmenger's complex

Q 42. The cardiovascular response to cooling to 31°C in a healthy 20-year-old is likely to include:

A. bradycardia
B. prolonged PR interval
C. prolonged QT interval
D. ventricular fibrillation
E. asystole

Q 43. In making a diagnosis of brain stem death:

A. the clinicians performing the tests must have been registered medical practitioners for at least three years
B. at least one clinician must be a consultant
C. the blood urea and electrolytes must be in the normal range

D. the legal time of death is after the first tests
E. the apnoea tests stipulates that the $PaCO_2$ must be greater than 5.6 kPa

Q 44. Tramadol:

A. blocks the release of 5-HT
B. must be given intravenously
C. may be used in patients on monoamine oxidase inhibitor (MAOI)
D. causes histamine release
E. is contraindicated in renal failure

Q 45. Concerning albumin:

A. the molecular size is approximately 90,000 daltons
B. approximately 9 to 12 g/day are synthesised by the average adult
C. serum levels are normally measured by immunoassay
D. is predominantly an intravascular protein
E. synthesis is initially increased as part of an acute phase response

Q 46. The group A antigen:

A. is carried by all the red cells of group A patients
B. is the most common cause of haemolytic disease of the new born
C. can occur in the saliva of group A patients
D. is transmitted according to Mendelian principles
E. is more common than group B antigen in Caucasians

Q 47. Disequilibrium during haemodialysis:

A. is more common in patients suffering from acute renal failure
B. can be treated with a glucose infusion
C. is less common with bicarbonate dialysis
D. is due to relative autonomic failure
E. may present as epileptiform fits

Q 48. A 65-year-old man is admitted in acute respiratory failure. Arterial blood gas results consistent with his condition, being an acute exacerbation of an underlying chronic obstructive airways disease with chronic bronchitis would include:

A. a $PaCO_2$ of 8.5 kPa
B. a PaO_2 of 11.5 kPa with an FiO_2 of 24%
C. an actual bicarbonate of 22 mmol/l
D. a haemoglobin of 12.6 g/dl
E. a pH of 7.45

Q 49. In patients with acute respiratory distress syndrome (ARDS):

A. high frequency ventilation is mandatory
B. methyl prednisolone 30 mg/kg is of proven benefit
C. an inverted inspiratory expiratory ratio is used to generate auto positive end expiratory pressure (PEEP)
D. it is essential to infuse albumin to maintain a normal colloid osmotic pressure
E. the preferred weaning mode includes continuous positive airway pressure (CPAP)

Q 50. Measurements of peak expiratory flow rate:

A. reveals a normal diurnal variation of less than 10%
B. is made approximately using a vitalograph
C. with a Wright peak flow meter uses the principle of a constant orifice with a variable pressure drop
D. can be achieved using a rapid capnograph
E. produces a reading, which is normally at 450–650 l/min in the adult

Q 51. Patients with acromegaly have:

A. sensitivity to insulin
B. a normal life expectancy
C. soft tissue hypertrophy of the pharyngeal mucosa
D. a basophil adenoma
E. increased risk of developing Conn's syndrome

Paper 3 Questions

Q 52. The carcinoid syndrome is associated with elevated levels of:

- **A.** epinephrine
- **B.** insulin
- **C.** glucagon
- **D.** prostaglandins
- **E.** serotonin

Q 53. Endotoxin:

- **A.** is usually found in patients suffering from sepsis syndrome
- **B.** may be degraded by the administration of antibiotics directed at the O antigen
- **C.** can be detected with a test using crab blood
- **D.** if injected into volunteers lowers pulmonary arterial pressure
- **E.** consists of two main components

Q 54. The following correlate with the severity and a poor outcome in acute pancreatitis:

- **A.** serum amylase activity
- **B.** plasma glucose concentration
- **C.** body mass index
- **D.** serum lactate dehydrogenase activity
- **E.** plasma C reactive protein

Q 55. The incidence if respiratory depression in patients receiving patient controlled analgesia is increased by:

- **A.** reducing the lockout time
- **B.** using a background infusion
- **C.** increasing the bolus dose
- **D.** concomitant non-steroidal anti-inflammatory drug (NSAID) administration
- **E.** concomitant sedative administration

Q 56. The crush syndrome:

- **A.** results from extensive tissue ischaemia
- **B.** is seen in compartment syndrome
- **C.** results in myoglobinuria

D. may require deliberate acidification of the urine to prevent renal failure
E. commonly causes disseminated intravascular coagulation

Q 57. Wind up is:

A. the augmented response to repetitive C fibre stimulation
B. associated with increased activity of second order neurones in the substantia gelatinosa
C. mediated by a glutamate receptors of the N-methyl D-aspartate (NMDA) subtype
D. can be reduced by morphine acting on the spinal cord
E. is blocked by intrathecal 5-HT_3 receptor agonist analogues

Q 58. An obstetrician calls urgently for help because a previous undiagnosed twin has been trapped in the uterus following the injection of ergometrine. The action of ergometrine can be reversed by:

A. salbutamol
B. ritodrine
C. isoflurane
D. thiopentone
E. suxamethonium

Q 59. Routine preoperative chest X-ray is indicated in:

A. those with possible metastases
B. every patient over 70 years
C. those with well controlled blood pressure
D. heavy smokers who have not had a previous chest X-ray
E. recent immigrants from countries where tuberculosis is endemic who have not had an X-ray within the previous 12 months

Q 60. The process of red cell transfusion:

A. the blood compatibility label must be checked to ensure that the blood is correct for the patient
B. the bag should be inspected to ensure integrity of the plastic casing
C. blood left out of the blood fridge for longer than 15 min should be discarded

D. the expiratory date should be checked
E. the volume of blood transfused should be recorded once administered

Q 61. A eutectic mixture of local anaesthetic:

A. can be formed by any local anaesthetic drug
B. contains 5% lidocaine and 5% prilocaine when formulated as EMLA cream
C. results from alteration in the melting point of the anaesthetic bases
D. can be formed from the carbonated salts of local anaesthetics
E. contains epinephrine

Q 62. In patients with established renal failure:

A. pericarditis is a complication
B. digoxin excretion is impaired
C. the elimination half-life of pancuronium is normal
D. acidosis aids reversal of non-depolarising relaxants
E. high dose diuretics improve the outcomes

Q 63. Features of Addison's disease include:

A. a benefit from ACTH
B. insulin resistance
C. an inability to excrete a water load
D. hypertension
E. hyperkalaemia

Q 64. Hepatitis C:

A. is a DNA virus
B. may be transmitted via blood products
C. usually presents as a flu like illness
D. rarely develops into chronic liver disease
E. leads to a full recovery in 20% of cases

Q 65. The following may result in haemoptysis:

A. mitral stenosis
B. Good Pasteur syndrome
C. Wegener's granulomatosis

D. Behçet's disease
E. bronchiectasis

Q 66. Perioperative management of a jaundiced patient should include:

A. mannitol infusion
B. a clotting screen
C. prophylactic antibiotics
D. intravenous vitamin K
E. thromboembolic prophylaxis with subcutaneous heparin

Q 67. A primary bronchogenic carcinoma is associated with:

A. diabetes insipidus
B. carcinoid syndrome
C. hypertrophic pulmonary osteoarthropathy
D. Horner's syndrome
E. thyrotoxicosis

Q 68. A patient had a traumatic quadriplegia after an accident 2 weeks ago. The likely problems include:

A. increased resistance to suxamethonium
B. urinary retention
C. adductor spasm of the legs
D. hyperthermia
E. intermittent positive pressure ventilation (IPPV) causes hypotension

Q 69. In a patient with dystrophia myotonica:

A. spinal anaesthesia produces muscular relaxation
B. suxamethonium has a normal effect
C. non-depolarising neuromuscular blocking drugs do not abolish the myotonia
D. non-depolarising neuromuscular blocking drugs produce an enhanced effect
E. diaphragmatic function is not affected

Q 70. In acute hepatic failure:

A. the prothrombin time is in excess of 20 s
B. serum alkaline phosphatase may be normal

C. albumin production is unaffected
D. plasma bilirubin is a sensitive indicator of hepatocellular damage
E. serum ADH is a sensitive indicator of hepatocellular damage

Q 71. The following cause hypokalaemic alkalosis:

A. prolonged vomiting
B. Cushing's diseases
C. frusemide
D. renal tubular acidosis
E. chronic renal failure

Q 72. The factors affecting the rate of transport of a drug across the placenta are the:

A. placental blood flow
B. degree of ionisation
C. degree of protein binding
D. pK of the drug
E. lipid solubility of the drug

Q 73. In radiation:

A. the SI unit of radioactivity is the curie
B. a γ-ray is an electromagnetic wave
C. an X-ray is a type of non-ionising radiation
D. the rate of decay of a radioactive substance is linear
E. γ-rays travel shorter distances than α or β particles

Q 74. Causes of respiratory distress in the neonate include:

A. unilateral choanal atresia
B. a tracheo-oesophageal fistula
C. a diaphragmatic hernia
D. necrotising enterocolitis
E. a myelomeningocoele

Q 75. The following are to be expected in a patient who is HIV positive and in whom a diagnosis of *Pneumocystis carinii* is suspected:

A. breathlessness
B. haemoptysis
C. pleuritic chest pain
D. pyrexia
E. a CD4 lymphocyte count of 2.4×10^9/l

Q 76. The volume occupied by one gram molecular weight of a gas:

A. varies directly with pressure
B. varies inversely with temperature
C. is related to its vapour density
D. is called the specific volume
E. is 22.4 l at room temperature for all gases

Q 77. Troponin I level in plasma:

A. rises with both ischaemia and infarction
B. is proportional to the amount of necrosis
C. is less sensitive than troponin T
D. peaks after CK
E. may offer enhanced specificity in patients with surgical skeletal muscle damage

Q 78. The following are the advantages of using glycine during TURP:

A. better optical conditions for the surgeon
B. when absorbed intravenously it is associated with less haemolysis than water
C. it is isotonic with plasma
D. it does not dissipate the cutting current
E. it is not absorbed systemically

Q 79. Student's t-test:

A. is used to compare small samples
B. does not require a null hypothesis

C. is a non-parametric test
D. is based on the t-distribution
E. is the most sensitive test for detecting a genuine difference

Q 80. The following ECG changes are consistent with acute myocardial infarction of 6 h duration:

A. Q waves in leads overlying the infarction
B. T wave inversion
C. ST segment elevation
D. S1, Q3, T3 pattern is usual
E. ST segment elevation, which persists, may indicate a ventricular aneurysm

Q 81. The following can be used to enhance endogenous antioxidant defences:

A. N-acetylcysteine
B. ascorbic acid (vitamin C)
C. albumin
D. dimethylsulphoxide
E. lazaroids

Q 82. The common presenting symptoms of an epidural abscess include:

A. backache
B. weakness of an extremity
C. bladder and bowel dysfunction
D. radicular pain
E. pyrexia

Q 83. The benefits of "off-pump" coronary artery surgery include:

A. a shorter time requiring ventilatory support
B. less blood loss
C. less need for blood transfusion
D. increased systemic inflammatory response
E. shorter hospital stay

Q 84. Drugs which have a context sensitive half-life, which increases with time, include:

- **A.** remifentanil
- **B.** alfentanil
- **C.** propofol
- **D.** morphine
- **E.** fentanyl

Q 85. Obesity:

- **A.** is an independent risk factor for ischaemic heart disease
- **B.** prolongs the elimination half life of thiopentone
- **C.** cause a fall in lung compliance
- **D.** is associated with a significant reduction in functional residual capacity and residual volume (RV)
- **E.** is associated with an increase in the glomerular filtration rate

Q 86. With regard to hepatic blood flow the following will decrease the flow:

- **A.** regional anaesthesia
- **B.** all inhalational anaesthetic agents
- **C.** halothane anaesthesia associated with hyperventilation
- **D.** intermittent positive pressure ventilation
- **E.** hypotension

Q 87. Complications of a subtotal thyroidectomy include:

- **A.** aphonia
- **B.** asphyxia
- **C.** recurrence of thyrotoxicosis
- **D.** myxoedema
- **E.** hypercalcaemia

Q 88. When considering drug therapy during pregnancy:

- **A.** methyldopa is contraindicated at all stages
- **B.** treatment with isotretinoin is a recognised indication for termination
- **C.** folic acid supplements should be given to patients taking phenytoin

D. thiazide diuretics have been shown to decrease placental perfusion
E. heparin has been shown to cause central nervous system damage in the foetus if given in the second and third trimesters

Q 89. Irritable bowel syndrome is associated with:

A. the passing of mucus per rectum
B. per rectal bleeding
C. abdominal pain relieved by defaecation
D. abdominal bloating
E. weight loss

Q 90. Heinz bodies may result from:

A. microangiopathic haemolytic anaemia
B. glucose-6-phosphate dehydrogenase deficiency
C. drug induced haemolysis
D. thalassaemia
E. sickle cell anaemia

Table for your Answers

Question	A	B	C	D	E
1					
2					
3					
4					
5					
6					
7					
8					
9					
10					
11					
12					
13					
14					
15					
16					
17					
18					
19					
20					
21					
22					
23					
24					
25					
26					
27					
28					
29					
30					

Paper 3

Questions

Question	A	B	C	D	E
31					
32					
33					
34					
35					
36					
37					
38					
39					
40					
41					
42					
43					
44					
45					
46					
47					
48					
49					
50					
51					
52					
53					
54					
55					
56					
57					
58					
59					
60					

Question	A	B	C	D	E
61					
62					
63					
64					
65					
66					
67					
68					
69					
70					
71					
72					
73					
74					
75					
76					
77					
78					
79					
80					
81					
82					
83					
84					
85					
86					
87					
88					
89					
90					

Paper 4 Questions

Q 1. The brachial plexus:

A. roots arise from C4 to T1
B. innervates serratus anterior
C. is in part accompanied by the subclavian artery
D. passes under the first rib
E. lies anterior to the perivascular sheath in the axilla

Q 2. In the management of paracetamol poisoning:

A. gastric lavage is indicated within 4 h of ingestion
B. pre-existing treatment with carbamazepine reduces the risk of liver damage
C. haemodialysis will enhance the clearance of paracetamol
D. acetyl cysteine is given to replenish intracellular glutamate
E. a plasma pH >7.5 is evidence of hepatocellular failure

Q 3. The effectiveness of defibrillation is increased by:

A. acidosis
B. class Ia anti-arrhythmic drugs
C. bretylium
D. delivery during inspiration
E. ensuring uniform distribution of the applied current within the heart

Q 4. Albumin:

A. is a branched polysaccharide with variable molecular weight
B. is the principle contributor to the colloid osmotic pressure of plasma
C. is widely distributed outside the circulation
D. is synthesised by haemopoetic stem cells
E. is present in normal urine

Q 5. In the treatment of ventricular arrhythmias intravenous lidocaine may be used safely in patients:

- **A.** hypersensitive to para-aminobenzoic acid
- **B.** hypersensitive to procaine
- **C.** with a permanent pacemaker
- **D.** with a history of epilepsy
- **E.** who are chronically digitalised

Q 6. Oxygen failure devices on anaesthetic machines require that:

- **A.** when activated the auditory alarm shall last 2 s
- **B.** the energy required to operate the alarm shall be derived solely from the oxygen supply pressure
- **C.** the alarm shall be activated when the oxygen supply pressure is halved
- **D.** when activated the flow of nitrous oxide shall be shut off
- **E.** when activated the oxygen flush function shall be maintained

Q 7. A 41-year-old lady weighing 65 kg is found to have carcinoma of the left lung. The following contraindicate lung resection:

- **A.** a history of haemoptysis
- **B.** ischaemic changes on the ECG
- **C.** recent onset of hoarseness
- **D.** an FEV1 of 2 l
- **E.** a vital capacity of less than 1,500 ml

Q 8. Patients with greater than normal risk of developing gram negative septicaemia include those suffering from:

- **A.** diabetes mellitus
- **B.** cirrhosis
- **C.** leukaemia
- **D.** uraemia
- **E.** polycythaemia

Q 9. The pathophysiological consequences of acute, severe asthma include:

- **A.** a predisposition to pulmonary oedema
- **B.** a decreased blood pressure

C. an increased biventricular after load
D. an increased alveolar ventilation
E. a focal myocardial necrosis

Q 10. Features of neurolept malignant syndrome include:

A. renal failure
B. temperature >40°C
C. lead pipe muscle rigidity
D. persistent neurological deficit
E. tachycardia and sweating

Q 11. The following drugs commonly used in intensive care should be given in reduced dosage in patients with renal impairment:

A. paracetamol
B. midazolam
C. cephalosporins
D. erythromycin
E. metronidazole

Q 12. Post herpetic neuralgia is:

A. much less severe after acute phase treatment with acyclovir
B. responsive to capsaicin induced A fibre desensitisation
C. caused by varicella zoster infection
D. associated with unpleasant skin sensitivity
E. treated with gasserian ganglion ablation

Q 13. Pulmonary capillary wedge pressure (PCPW) is greater than left ventricular end diastolic pressure (LVEDP) in the following circumstances:

A. mitral stenosis
B. pulmonary embolism
C. a catheter wedged in the upper zone of the lung
D. a normal patient in the supine position
E. severe left ventricular failure

Q 14. The blood-brain barrier:

A. is composed mainly of endothelial cells
B. restricts passive diffusion of glucose from blood to brain

C. is functionally affected by CNS infection
D. is less permeable in neonates than in adults
E. restricts passive diffusion of lipophilic drugs from blood to brain

Q 15. When performing the three-in-one block for pain relief in lower limb surgery:

A. the needle is inserted medial to the femoral artery
B. the saphenous nerve will be blocked
C. good analgesia will be obtained for operations on the foot
D. the obturator nerve, femoral nerve and the lateral cutaneous nerves of the thigh will be blocked
E. muscle relaxation is provided

Q 16. A man aged 35 years who has suffered from asthma suddenly becomes increasingly breathless. The following investigations are particularly useful:

A. serum glucose
B. eosinophil count
C. clinical examination of the sputum
D. ECG
E. peak expiratory flow rate

Q 17. The following scoring systems are commonly used in the critically ill to assess disease severity:

A. Sepsis related oxygen failure assessment (SOFA)
B. Therapeutic intervention scoring system (TISS)
C. Simplified acute physiological score (SAPS)
D. Glasgow coma score (GCS)
E. Ramsey score

Q 18. The indications for routine preoperative urea and electrolytes include:

A. all patients over 70
B. those with a history of renal disease
C. those on diuretic therapy
D. all major operations
E. those with a history of diarrhoea and vomiting

Paper 4 Questions

Q 19. The routine management of all patients in the recovery room includes the monitoring of the:

A. level of consciousness
B. haemoglobin oxygen saturation and oxygen administration
C. blood pressure
D. respiratory frequency
E. pain intensity by verbal rating scale

Q 20. The pudendal nerve block provides analgesia to the:

A. cervix
B. peroneal body
C. labia minora
D. labia majora
E. anterior vaginal wall

Q 21. The amino acid glutamate is:

A. an essential amino acid
B. used as an energy source by enterocytes
C. used as an energy source by polymorph-nuclear leukocytes
D. stable in solution
E. the sulphydryl donor of reduced glutathione

Q 22. The TEC 5 vaporiser:

A. is non-spill at an angle of 180°
B. has the thermostat in the vaporising chamber
C. has the same capacity as a TEC 4
D. delivers isoflurane at a constant concentration over 15 min when the dial is set at 4%
E. has a greater wick area than that of the TEC 4

Q 23. Patients with chronic alcoholism are likely to demonstrate:

A. a high MAC for enflurane
B. a prolonged anaesthetic induction time
C. resistance to the hypnotic effect of thiopentone
D. arterial hypoxaemia
E. resistance to non-depolarising neuromuscular blockade

Q 24. The operation of the standard cylinder pressure gauge is based on the:

A. Hagen-Poiseuille law
B. Fixed orifice principle
C. Bernoulli principle
D. Bourdon tube principle
E. Critical flow rate principle

Q 25. An acutely developing blood coagulation defect associated with massive transfusion may be due to:

A. disseminated intravascular coagulation (DIC)
B. thrombocytopenia
C. deficiency of clotting factor V and VIII
D. a transfusion reaction
E. fibrinolysis

Q 26. In a previously well-controlled insulin dependent diabetic, insulin requirements increase:

A. in the third trimester of pregnancy
B. in thyrotoxicosis
C. in chronic renal failure
D. after pituitary ablation for retinopathy
E. if given with propranolol

Q 27. Phosphate:

A. ions are the most abundant intracellular anion
B. in blood the majority of phosphate is in the inorganic form
C. absorption from the gut is enhanced by calcitonin
D. in serum of less than 1.2 mmol/l indicates hypophosphataemia
E. rapid correction of hypophosphataemia causes central pontine myelinosis

Q 28. Carboxyhaemoglobin:

A. blood levels of 20% or more are found in smokers
B. has an affinity for haemoglobin 150 times greater than oxygen

C. displaces the oxygen dissociation curve to the left
D. has a half-life of 4 h in patients breathing room air
E. has a half-life of less than 20 min in patients breathing 100% oxygen

Q 29. Non-steroidal anti-inflammatory drugs (NSAIDs):

A. are effective as the sole analgesic agent after major surgery
B. interact with cyclosporins
C. exert their analgesia effect by inhibition of cyclo-oxygenase (COX)
D. can be used in patients with aspirin sensitive asthma
E. increase bleeding

Q 30. Hyperparathyroidism is associated with:

A. a rise in calcitonin levels
B. an increase in urinary phosphate excretion
C. osteitis fibrosis cystica
D. hypercalcaemia
E. low urinary calcium

Q 31. Traumatic rupture of the thoracic aorta is associated with:

A. a history of penetrating injury of the chest
B. fracture of the upper ribs
C. widening of the mediastinum
D. deviation of the naso-gastric tube to the left
E. elevation of the left main bronchus

Q 32. A patient taking a monoamine oxidase inhibitor (MAOI) presents for elective cholecystectomy. The anaesthetic management should include:

A. premedication with 400 μg/kg hyoscine
B. preloading with 500 ml of 0.9% normal saline
C. epidural analgesia with 0.5% bupivacaine
D. general anaesthesia with thiopentone, vecuronium, oxygen and isoflurane
E. subcutaneous heparin

Q 33. Likely causes of surgical emphysema in patients with vomiting and abdominal pain and dyspepsia include:

A. ruptured trachea
B. ruptured oesophagus
C. spontaneous pneumothorax
D. pulmonary embolism
E. ruptured larynx

Q 34. Symptoms of hyperthyroidism likely to occur in a 25-year-old women include:

A. cold intolerance
B. reduced pulse pressure
C. lid lag
D. menorrhagia
E. a thyroid bruit

Q 35. Characteristic features of overdose of a tricyclic antidepressant include:

A. meiosis
B. tachycardia
C. urinary retention
D. skin changes
E. metabolic acidosis

Q 36. Concerning cerebral protection:

A. Thiopentone reduces cerebral oxygen consumption by up to 60%
B. Thiopentone is ineffective if the insult is due to cardiac arrest
C. The effectiveness of thiopentone is due to a reduction in cerebral blood flow
D. Thiopentone is more effective if given before the insult
E. Calcium channel blockers are effective

Q 37. Blood gas analysers directly measure:

A. PaO_2
B. oxygen content
C. base excess

D. bicarbonate concentration
E. atmospheric pressure

Q 38. The following are included in Child's classification of liver failure:

A. plasma albumin concentration
B. plasma bilirubin concentration
C. the degree of ascites
D. prothrombin time
E. the nutritional state of the patient

Q 39. To perform carotid endarterectomy under local anaesthesia the following nerves should be blocked:

A. lesser occipital nerve
B. facial nerve
C. transverse cervical nerve
D. lesser auricular nerve
E. subscapular nerve

Q 40. Diamorphine as compared to morphine:

A. has a faster onset of action
B. decreased delayed respiratory depression when administered intrathecally
C. has no active metabolites
D. 20 mg is roughly equivalent to 20 mg oxycodone
E. has a high first pass metabolism

Q 41. A 3-year-old child with a history of wheeze for 3 days which is unresponsive to a salbutamol inhaler, is cyanosed and restless with PaO_2 4.5 kPa and $PaCO_2$ 9 kPa, should have, as a primary line of treatment:

A. intravenous aminophylline
B. intravenous bicarbonate
C. immediate intubation and ventilation
D. intravenous midazolam
E. sodium chromoglycate

Q 42. In epiglottitis the following are true:

A. iv access should come first
B. immediate lateral neck X-ray will aid diagnosis

C. iv chloramphenicol is the treatment of choice
D. the patient is likely to be intubated for 5 days
E. tracheotomy should be performed if the patient is still intubated after 72 h

Q 43. In patients in whom the diagnosis of multiple sclerosis is to be considered:

A. abnormal visual evoked responses are diagnostic
B. an absent deep tendon reflex excludes the diagnosis
C. the absence of sensory signs makes the diagnosis unlikely
D. the disease is excluded if there is no history of measles
E. rapidly progressive neurological deficit excludes the diagnosis

Q 44. The following are contraindications to perform a magnetic resonance scan:

A. dental fillings
B. a posterior communicating aneurysm clipped three years ago
C. a cardiac pacemaker
D. a Starr Edward's prosthetic cardiac valve
E. a hip prosthesis

Q 45. The following reliably indicate that an episode of transient cerebral ischaemia is in the territory of the carotid artery:

A. monocular visual loss
B. hemianopia
C. diplopia
D. dysphonia
E. unilateral facial and arm sensory loss

Q 46. Constrictive pericarditis is secondary to:

A. tuberculosis
B. myocardial infarction
C. *Staphylococcus aureus* infection
D. uraemia
E. coxsakie B virus infection

Q 47. Cold cardioplegic solutions:

A. are usually at 10°C
B. may contain amino acids

C. usually contain more than 25 mmol/l of potassium
D. are used to arrest the heart diastole
E. are delivered via the coronary sinus

Q 48. Dopexamine:

A. has no α_1-adrenergic agonist activity
B. has active metabolites which are excreted in urine
C. has little β_2-adrenergic agonist activity
D. is actively taken up by sympathetic nerves
E. inhibits the neuronal re-uptake of noradrenaline

Q 49. Patients with HELLP syndrome:

A. always have a thrombocytopenia
B. usually have pre-eclampsia
C. usually have a normal APTT
D. can present post-partum
E. should not have an epidural regional block

Q 50. Verapamil:

A. decreases calcium entry into the mitochondria
B. decreases the QT interval
C. delays conduction at the AV node
D. delays excretion of digoxin
E. may safely be co-administered with a β-blocker

Q 51. Recognised manifestations of carbon monoxide poisoning include:

A. nausea and vomiting
B. intellectual impairment in survivors
C. cerebral signs
D. bullous skin lesions
E. left shift of the oxygen dissociation curve

Q 52. Air embolism during surgery is dangerous because:

A. a patent foramen ovale is present in 15% of the population
B. air can pass through the bronchial vessels to the systemic circulation
C. air can obstruct the coronary vessels

D. it causes a rise in pulmonary artery resistance and pressure
E. ventricular fibrillation may occur

Q 53. The following are examples of resistance transducers:

A. Condenser microphone
B. Thermocouple
C. Strain gauge
D. Thermistor
E. Piezoelectric crystals

Q 54. Glycolysis:

A. is the breakdown of glucose to pyruvic acid or lactate
B. releases energy to be utilised by the production of ADP
C. under anaerobic conditions pyruvic acid enters the Kreb's (TCA) cycle with a net gain of 38 moles of ATP
D. under anaerobic conditions the net gain of ATP is 2 moles per mole of glucose
E. occurs in red cells and exercising muscle

Q 55. The following are risk factors for postoperative stroke in the elderly:

A. hypertension
B. physical inactivity
C. atherosclerosis
D. haemodynamic instability
E. major intraoperative blood loss

Q 56. In variant Creutzfeldt-Jakob disease:

A. the infective agents appear to be misshapen prion protein
B. the infectious agent is resistant to methods of sterilisation currently used
C. in the UK, a sporadic form of the disease of unknown cause is responsible for 73% of cases
D. a familial form is associated with a single gene mutation
E. prion expression in lympho-reticular tissue appears to occur from a very early stage of the disease

Paper 4

Questions

Q 57. The following are pro-inflammatory cytokines:

A. TNF-α
B. IL-10
C. IL-6
D. IL-1
E. Granuloctye colony stimulation factor

Q 58. Cocaine:

A. is a directly acting sympathomimetic
B. when administered topically should not exceed a dose of 3 mg/kg
C. offers no advantage over lignocaine topically
D. overdose should be treated with α and β antagonists
E. has an intrinsic vasoconstrictor activity

Q 59. The following clinical and laboratory features are helpful in the diagnosis of fat embolism:

A. an elevated erythrocyte sedimentation rate (ESR)
B. fat macroglobulinaemia
C. thrombocytosis
D. petechial rash
E. early hypoxaemia

Q 60. Classical haemophilia (factor VIII deficiency):

A. is associated with a positive family history in at least 90% of cases
B. never occurs in the female
C. is associated with a normal bleeding time
D. usually presents with a gastrointestinal haemorrhage
E. can be successfully treated by the infusion of banked plasma

Q 61. Appropriate treatment of grand mal seizures occurring after surgical removal of a cortical meningioma include:

A. intravenous mannitol
B. intravenous phenytoin
C. intravenous thiopentone infusion
D. intravenous clonazepam
E. hyperventilation

Q 62. Hepatic encephalopathy in a patient with liver disease can be precipitated by:

A. constipation
B. bleeding from a duodenal ulcer
C. surgery
D. barbiturates
E. oral neomycin

Q 63. The following may be associated with insertion of Harrington rods in spinal surgery:

A. upper gastrointestinal obstruction
B. spinal cord ischaemia
C. fat embolism
D. hypothermia
E. pneumothorax

Q 64. Following thiopentone induction, blood pressure falls to 60/40 mmHg and the heart rate increases from 60 to 72 bpm. Isoprenaline would be useful if the patient had:

A. severe aortic stenosis
B. severe mitral stenosis
C. ischaemic heart disease
D. chronic mitral regurgitation
E. tetralogy of Fallot

Q 65. Magnesium sulphate used in the management of pre-eclampsia and eclampsia:

A. reduces the excitability of the skeletal muscle membrane
B. decreases acetylcholine release at the neuromuscular junction
C. is antagonised by intravenous calcium chloride
D. is excreted almost entirely by the kidney
E. produces myocardial depression

Q 66. Concerning the anatomy of peripheral nerves:

A. The lumbar plexus is derived from T12 to L4
B. The cervical plexus is derived from C1, C2 and C3 spinal nerves

C. The femoral nerve supplies the skin over the anterior aspect of the thigh
D. The posterior tibial nerve is located between the lateral malleolus and the Achilles tendon
E. The peroneal nerves (superficial and deep) supply the dorsum of the foot

Q 67. At extubation following inadvertent left recurrent laryngeal nerve section during radical thyroidectomy, laryngoscopy would demonstrate the left vocal cord to be:

A. immobile
B. slack
C. hyperaemic
D. fully adducted
E. drawn towards the right cord on inspiration

Q 68. The following are likely to occur after injection of 10 units of syntocinon iv:

A. decreased systolic and diastolic blood pressure
B. skin vasodilatation
C. decreased systemic vascular resistance
D. reflex tachycardia
E. decreased cardiac output

Q 69. Ulcerative colitis is associated with:

A. uveitis
B. liver cirrhosis
C. cholangitis
D. clubbing
E. arthritis

Q 70. Post-dural puncture headache:

A. is relieved by lying flat
B. may be accompanied by meningism
C. mental depression is common
D. can appear at any time up to five days after dural puncture
E. cranial nerve palsies can develop particularly in nerves controlling eye movement

Q 71. The following drugs alter the level of thyroxine production:

A. amiodarone
B. propylthiouracil
C. propranolol
D. carbidopa
E. thymoxamine

Q 72. The following are correct:

A. 500 ml of 5% glucose contains 250 g of glucose
B. 40 ml of 0.5% prilocaine contains 100 mg prilocaine
C. 1 ml of 1:10,000 adrenaline contains 100 μg adrenaline
D. 10 ml of 1.0% lidocaine contains 100 mg lidocaine
E. 100 ml 8.4% sodium bicarbonate solution contains 100 mmol sodium bicarbonate

Q 73. The following are useful in the treatment of digitalis induced cardiac arrhythmias:

A. phenytoin
B. lidocaine
C. propranolol
D. potassium
E. procainamide

Q 74. Demonstration of the cerebral vessels surrounding a tumour by angiography under a general anaesthetic is improved by:

A. a 20% fall in mean systemic arterial pressure
B. a reduction of arterial oxygen tension to 8.0 kPa (60 mmHg)
C. a reduction of arterial carbon dioxide tension to 4.0 kPa (30 mmHg)
D. a rise in intracranial pressure to 13 kPa (100 mmHg)
E. assumption of the prone position

Q 75. General anaesthesia for elective major surgery is contraindicated in patients:

A. who have acute intermittent porphyria
B. who have congestive cardiac failure

C. with sickle cell disease
D. with an acute febrile upper respiratory tract infection
E. with a proven susceptibility to malignant hyperpyrexia

Q 76. During mechanical ventilation:

A. right atrial filling pressure increases
B. left atrial filling pressure rises
C. mean pleural pressure is unchanged
D. right ventricular afterload is reduced
E. left ventricular afterload is reduced

Q 77. The development of postoperative hypoglycaemia in a diabetic patient after amputation of an infected foot can result from:

A. the decreased insulin requirement after amputation
B. the stress response to surgery with release of glucagon
C. the effect of protamine zinc insulin given 24 h before operation
D. septicaemia
E. associated hypothermia

Q 78. Cardioversion:

A. can be performed without general anaesthesia
B. is safer using AC current than DC current
C. DC shock should be given at the upstroke of the Q wave
D. may cause ventricular fibrillation
E. is contraindicated in digitalised patients

Q 79. In disseminating intravascular coagulopathy:

A. the prothrombin time is normal
B. a low fibrinogen level is an indication for treatment with tranexamic acid
C. there is a micro capillary thrombosis
D. there is a primary fibrinolysis
E. tissue factor and cytokines are released from monocytes

Q 80. Venous air embolism is associated with:

A. arterial hypotension
B. a decrease in end-expiratory carbon dioxide concentration

C. cardiac arrhythmias
D. a decrease in pulmonary vascular resistance
E. an increase in intracranial pressure

Q 81. Muscle relaxation under intravenous regional anaesthesia (IVRA) may be enhanced by:

A. administration of 15 ml of 0.9% sodium chloride after the injection of the local anaesthetic
B. five minutes of pre-injection tourniquet ischaemia
C. using 1% procaine instead of 0.5% lidocaine
D. adding 3 mg alcuronium to the local anaesthesia
E. addition of adrenaline to the local anaesthetic

Q 82. Important landmarks to blockade of the median nerve at the elbow include the:

A. basilic vein
B. olecranon process
C. medial head of the triceps
D. brachial artery
E. cephalic vein

Q 83. In the new-born, a decrease in body temperature is accompanied by:

A. increased oxygen consumption
B. systemic arterial hypertension
C. metabolic alkalosis
D. hyper irritability
E. shivering

Q 84. Concerning a vapouriser for use inside the circle system:

A. it must be temperature compensated
B. it is better situated on the inspiratory limb
C. its internal volume must be greater than the patient's tidal volume
D. accurate calibration is essential
E. it should be capable of delivering high concentrations of anaesthetic vapour

Q 85. A drug, which acts rapidly on the central nervous system and has high plasma clearance will:

A. have a long terminal half-life
B. produce a bolus effect
C. be rapidly soluble in aqueous solution at pH 7
D. be rapidly excreted unchanged by the kidneys
E. have a large volume of distribution

Q 86. Isoflurane:

A. is a respiratory depressant
B. causes tachycardia
C. is associated with the development of convulsions
D. causes a dose related depression in systemic vascular resistance
E. is metabolised to inorganic fluoride ions

Q 87. Autonomic hyper-reflexia following spinal cord transection:

A. occurs most frequently at T6
B. is usually manifested by hypertension and bradycardia
C. results in vasodilatation above the level of injury
D. can lead to cerebral haemorrhage
E. results from a loss of inhibitory control from higher centres

Q 88. Macrocytosis with normoblastic bone marrow is a feature of:

A. pregnancy
B. chronic hepatitis
C. coeliac disease
D. thyroid disease
E. phenytoin administration

Q 89. The characteristic features of organophosphate poisoning include:

A. dilated pupils
B. rhinorrhoea
C. hyperventilation
D. muscle fasciculation
E. convulsions

Q 90. When acclimatising to life at high altitude:

A. the mean corpuscular haemoglobin concentration (MCHC) is increased
B. respiration becomes periodic
C. cardiac output is increased
D. pulmonary diffusion capacity decreases
E. airway resistance is decreased

Table for your Answers

Question	A	B	C	D	E
1					
2					
3					
4					
5					
6					
7					
8					
9					
10					
11					
12					
13					
14					
15					
16					
17					
18					
19					
20					
21					
22					
23					
24					
25					
26					
27					
28					
29					
30					

Question	A	B	C	D	E
31					
32					
33					
34					
35					
36					
37					
38					
39					
40					
41					
42					
43					
44					
45					
46					
47					
48					
49					
50					
51					
52					
53					
54					
55					
56					
57					
58					
59					
60					

Paper 4

Questions

Question	A	B	C	D	E
61					
62					
63					
64					
65					
66					
67					
68					
69					
70					
71					
72					
73					
74					
75					
76					
77					
78					
79					
80					
81					
82					
83					
84					
85					
86					
87					
88					
89					
90					

Paper 5 Questions

Q 1. In Guillain-Barré syndrome:

A. a preceding history of diarrhoea is a good prognostic sign
B. desaturation occurs early
C. the cerebrospinal fluid (CSF) shows a marked increase in white cell count
D. high dose steroids should start early
E. denervated muscles are usually pain free

Q 2. Acute respiratory distress syndrome (ARDS) is characterised by:

A. an increased mortality over the last decade
B. a better outcome if the normal arterial blood gases are achieved
C. radiological evidence of patchy infiltration
D. refractory hypoxaemia
E. reduced lung compliance

Q 3. Concerning the development of gram negative septic shock:

A. Circulating endotoxin causes the release of chemical mediators which increase vascular permeability
B. Lack of ATP results in failure of the sodium pump
C. Septicaemia results from instrumentation of the biliary tree
D. The fibrinolytic system in not involved
E. Steroids maintain the stability of lysosomal membrane

Q 4. Pharmacological agents used to decrease left ventricular afterload in a patient with an acute myocardial infarction include:

A. nitroglycerin
B. sodium nitroprusside
C. phentolamine

Paper 5 Questions

D. isoprenaline
E. nifedipine

Q 5. **Total body water is increased in adults on continuous positive pressure ventilation as a result of:**

A. decreased renal cortical blood flow
B. increased renal medullary blood flow
C. decreased cardiac output
D. increased central venous pressure
E. inhibition of atrial natriuretic peptide release

Q 6. **Neonates compared with adults are resistant to suxamethonium because:**

A. pseudocholinesterase is 50% more active in neonates
B. neonates have more motor end-plates per kg
C. suxamethonium is excreted by the neonate
D. neonates have a larger extracellular space per kg
E. neonates have a greater proportion of haemoglobin F

Q 7. **In Paget's disease:**

A. urinary calcium is increased
B. alkaline phosphates is increased
C. sarcomata are more frequent
D. spontaneous fractures heal poorly
E. bone blood flow may represent 20% of cardiac output at rest

Q 8. **The conventional oxygen fail-safe mechanism of anaesthetic machines:**

A. is pressure sensitive
B. eliminates the possibility of the patient becoming hypoxic
C. cuts off gas flows when activated
D. is flow sensitive
E. depends upon an intact electrical supply to the machine

Q 9. **In a circle breathing system:**

A. the capacity of the soda lime container should equal the patient's ideal tidal volume
B. adequate function can be obtained with one uni-directional valve

C. the adjustable relief valve is best situated between the patient and the soda lime container
D. the size of the reservoir bag is not critical
E. any vaporiser included in the circuit should be placed between the fresh gas inlet and the patient

Q 10. **Following tricycle overdose:**

A. blood levels of the drug accurately reflect the amount ingested
B. coma is an early feature
C. forced alkaline diuresis is indicated
D. there is a risk of cardiac ventricular conduction defects
E. instillation of activated charcoal is only indicated in the first 4 h after ingestion

Q 11. **Anaesthesia is induced and maintained in an adult by breathing 30% oxygen, 70% nitrous oxide and a volatile agent. The uptake of the nitrous oxide into the blood stream:**

A. exceeds 1 l/min during the first minute
B. is likely to exceed the uptake of the oxygen after 1 h of anaesthesia
C. is less than the amount of expired nitrogen during the first few minutes
D. is proportional to the difference between inspired and end-tidal PN_2O provided ventilation is constant
E. still occurs after 12 h of anaesthesia

Q 12. **Factors in acute renal failure that suggest an intrinsic cause include:**

A. urine osmolarity less than 400 mosmol/l
B. urine sodium concentration less than 30 mmol/l
C. proteinuria
D. urine/plasma creatinine ratio greater than 40
E. elevated urine glucose concentration

Q 13. **Transcutaneous electrical nerve stimulation (TENS):**

A. activates A δ fibres
B. involves low frequency, high intensity stimulation

C. activates fibres in the substantia gelatinosa
D. is effective in approximately 50% of patients with chronic back pain
E. usefully modifies stage 1 labour pain

Q 14. The oesophageal Doppler monitor:

A. measures blood flow velocity in the ascending thoracic aorta
B. uses an estimate of aortic cross sectional area derived from the patient's age, height and weight
C. reflects qualitative changes in the pulmonary artery occlusion pressures by changes in the corrected systolic flow time
D. is reliable when used with the inter-aortic balloon pump
E. can calculate the stroke volume and cardiac output

Q 15. When monitoring the electroencephalogram (EEG) with increasing depth of anaesthesia:

A. a shift in power towards the lower frequencies occurs
B. the spectral edge frequency increases
C. the amount of EEG suppression is independent of the volatile agent, if used at MAC equivalent dosage
D. bispectral analysis includes an estimate of phase coupling in multivariant analysis
E. the spectral edge frequency (SEF) 50 is equal to the median frequency

Q 16. After placement of a pulmonary artery flotation catheter, the following can be measured directly or derived:

A. oxygen consumption VO_2 (ml/min)
B. systemic vascular resistance index (SVRI)
C. pulmonary venous admixture or shunt fraction (Q_S/Q_T)
D. left ventricular stroke work index
E. left ventricular end diastolic volume

Q 17. Appropriate management of a female patient with untreated thyrotoxicosis requiring repair of an incarcerated femoral hernia includes:

A. intravenous propranolol
B. intravenous carbimazole
C. spinal anaesthesia

D. atropine premedication
E. intravenous chlorpromazine

Q 18. Potential complications of the use of neuromuscular blocking agents in the critically ill include:

A. cardiac arrhythmias
B. critical illness neuropathy
C. venous thromboembolism
D. peripheral nerve injury
E. protracted muscle weakness

Q 19. Indications for preoperative ECG include:

A. all patients over 50 years old
B. those with a history of heart disease
C. hypertension
D. those with a history of chronic obstructive airway disease (COAD)
E. patients with clinical signs of anaemia

Q 20. The current guidelines for transfusion of red cells include:

A. healthy patients should not be transfused if their haemoglobin is above 10 g/dl
B. a haemoglobin concentration between 8 and 10 g/dl is a safe level even for those patients with significant cardio-respiratory disease
C. symptomatic patients should be transfused
D. a haemoglobin concentration below 7 g/dl is a strong indication for transfusion
E. transfusion will become essential when the haemoglobin decreases to 5 g/dl

Q 21. Concerning the safe use and disposal of sharps:

A. Sharps must not be transferred between personnel and handling should be kept to a minimum
B. Blunt aspirating needles should be used for drawing up drugs
C. Needles should not be recapped or resheathed
D. Needles and syringes must not be dissembled by hand prior to disposal
E. In UK 25% of occupational injuries occurring in hospitals are attributed to sharp injuries

Paper 5 Questions

Q 22. Vertebro-basilar insufficiency can cause:

A. dizziness
B. weakness in the legs
C. dysphonia
D. dysphasia
E. dysarthria

Q 23. The pneomotachograph:

A. directly measures pressure changes across a resistance
B. must have a resistance of sufficient diameter to ensure laminar flow
C. is not suitable for accurate breath-by-breath monitoring
D. possess accuracy affected by temperature changes
E. possess accuracy unaffected by alterations in gas compositions

Q 24. Hepatitis B infection:

A. is transmitted by droplets
B. is highly contagious
C. is common in intravenous drug users
D. can be prevented by immunisation
E. predisposes to carcinoma of the liver

Q 25. The end tidal partial pressure of carbon dioxide:

A. exceeds the arterial PCO_2 if the patient is in the prone position
B. may be over-estimated if measured by infrared absorption in the presence of nitrous oxide
C. may be over-estimated if measured by mass spectrometry in the presence of nitrous oxide
D. during intermittent positive pressure ventilation (IPPV) will be a more accurate estimate of arterial PCO_2 if positive end expiratory pressure is applied
E. may be under-estimated if measured by mass spectrometry in the presence of water vapour

Q 26. Remifentanil:

A. is a piperidine derivative
B. does not cause muscle rigidity

C. has a quick offset of action due to its large volume of distribution
D. has a prolonged duration of action in patients with suxamethonium apnoea
E. undergoes extensive first pass metabolism in the lung

Q 27. An abnormal hypertensive response to ephedrine can occur with:

A. propranolol
B. monoamine oxidase inhibitors (MAOI)
C. levodopa
D. fluoxetine
E. carbamazepine

Q 28. When magnesium sulphate is used in the treatment of pregnancy-induced hypertension:

A. acetylcholine release is reduced
B. most is eliminated via the kidney
C. its action is antagonised by iv calcium chloride
D. it leads to myocardial depression
E. it leads to convulsions

Q 29. The following are indications for hyperbaric oxygen therapy:

A. narcotising soft tissue infections
B. progressive myopia
C. decompression sickness
D. clostridia infections
E. carbon monoxide poisoning

Q 30. Diffusion capacity (Transfer factor):

A. is the rate of CO transfer per mmHg pressure difference between alveolar gas and pulmonary capillary blood
B. transfer is diffusion limited
C. is measured after a deep inspiration of 20% CO and 10 s breath hold
D. is normally 30 ml/min/mmHg
E. can be corrected for lung volume by dividing DLCO by FRC

Q 31. Serum electrolyte measurements of sodium 127 mmol/l and potassium 6.1 mmol/l are consistent with a diagnosis of:

A. acute renal failure
B. hypopituitarism
C. Addison's disease
D. primary hyperaldosteronism
E. Cushing's disease

Q 32. The following decrease intraocular pressure:

A. hypocapnia
B. hypoxia
C. enflurane
D. etomidate
E. non-depolarising muscle relaxants

Q 33. Physical signs found in pure mitral stenosis include:

A. a displaced apex beat
B. a sharp rising carotid up stroke
C. an accentuated first heart sound
D. an early diastolic murmur
E. presystolic accentuation of a diastolic murmur

Q 34. Features typical of injury to the radial nerve include:

A. inability to extend the elbow
B. wrist drop
C. anaesthesia over the base of the thumb
D. claw hand
E. inability to pronate the forearm

Q 35. The following physical signs are characteristic of pulmonary embolism:

A. dyspnoea
B. a large "a" wave on the jugular venous pressure (JVP)
C. raised systolic blood pressure
D. cyanosis
E. triple apex rhythm

Q 36. Post herpetic neuralgia:

- **A.** is more common above the age of 70
- **B.** is more common in men
- **C.** is frequently unilateral
- **D.** affects the nerve fibres equally within the nerve trunk
- **E.** is treated with rhizotomy

Q 37. Ropivacaine:

- **A.** is a propyl homologue of bupivacaine
- **B.** is 95% protein bound
- **C.** has the same relative toxicity as bupivacaine although cardiac side effects are more likely
- **D.** causes local vasoconstriction
- **E.** maximum safe dose is 2 mg/kg

Q 38. Amiodarone:

- **A.** slows conduction velocity in the Hiss-Purkinjee system
- **B.** prolongs the action potential duration in the SA node
- **C.** prolongs repolarisation in the AV node
- **D.** may cause photosensitivity
- **E.** may alter thyroid function tests

Q 39. The effects of moving from sea level to an altitude of 5,000 m include:

- **A.** alveolar PO_2 nearly reaches PO_2 in air
- **B.** increased plasma volume
- **C.** reduced blood bicarbonate level
- **D.** reduced exercise tolerance
- **E.** increased alveolar ventilation due to central chemoreceptor stimulation

Q 40. In a phaeochromocytoma treated with α-blockers there is:

- **A.** decreased systolic blood pressure
- **B.** decreased heart rate
- **C.** miosis
- **D.** cold peripheries
- **E.** postural hypotension

Q 41. Cyanosis at birth occurs in:

- **A.** tetralogy of Fallot
- **B.** transposition of the great vessels
- **C.** pulmonary stenosis (isolated)
- **D.** patent ductus arteriosus
- **E.** ventricular septal defect

Q 42. The development of anti-D antibodies in an Rh-negative mother with an Rh-positive baby is associated with:

- **A.** transfer of red cells from the baby to the mother
- **B.** an anaemic baby
- **C.** a jaundiced baby
- **D.** the passage of antigen from baby to mother
- **E.** the last trimester only

Q 43. A leaking aortic aneurysm can present with:

- **A.** severe abdominal pain
- **B.** hypotension
- **C.** anuria
- **D.** bruising in the loins
- **E.** absent femoral pulses

Q 44. The following are characteristic of polymyalgia rheumatica:

- **A.** proximal muscle wasting
- **B.** muscle tenderness
- **C.** pyrexia
- **D.** weight loss
- **E.** jaw claudication

Q 45. In tetanus:

- **A.** the longer the incubation period the more severe is the disease
- **B.** the diagnosis must be confirmed by isolation of *Clostridium tetani* from the wound
- **C.** respiratory muscle spasms leading to respiratory failure is a recognised cause of death

D. human anti-tetanus immunoglobulin cannot remove the toxin once it has been taken up from the blood into the peripheral nerve
E. a clinical attack confers immunity

Q 46. Plummer Vincent syndrome is associated with:

A. a pharyngeal pouch
B. ulcerative colitis
C. megaloblastic anaemia
D. dysphagia
E. iron deficiency anaemia

Q 47. Therapeutic administration of aprotinin:

A. inhibits kallikrein
B. may cause anaphylaxis
C. inhibits trypsin and plasmin
D. enhances platelet aggregation
E. should be monitored by repeated measurements of the ACT

Q 48. In sickle cell disease:

A. at least 50% of the red cell haemoglobin is in the foetal form (HbF)
B. diactylitis is an early sign in infancy
C. splenomegaly is a characteristic sign in adults
D. iron therapy is valuable if the patient is anaemic
E. travel in an unpressurised aircraft may precipitate a sickling crisis

Q 49. Inadequate analgesia over the radial artery during brachial plexus block can be due to failure to block the:

A. radial nerve
B. medial cutaneous nerve
C. musculocutaneous nerve
D. median nerve
E. ulnar nerve

Q 50. Intraoperative techniques for maintaining core temperature include:

A. use of warmed cotton blankets
B. use of warmed water mattresses
C. warmed iv fluids
D. forced air warming
E. heated and humidified inspired gases

Q 51. The following tests are recommended in the assessment of the patient with Parkinson's disease:

A. chest X-ray
B. pulmonary function tests
C. ECG
D. skin test energy
E. serum albumin

Q 52. Antithrombin III (AT III):

A. has a biological half-life of 7 to 9 days
B. is produced at a relatively constant rate
C. is not an acute phase respondent
D. normal range for AT III in plasma is based on a comparison with pooled plasma and is quoted as 50 to 90%
E. deficiency is associated with a decreased risk of thromboembolic disease

Q 53. The differential diagnosis of postpartum seizures include:

A. epilepsy
B. drug or alcohol withdraw
C. meningitis
D. an intracranial space occupying lesion
E. thrombotic thrombocytopenic purpura

Q 54. Concerning the meningococcus:

A. *Neisseria meningitidis* is an encapsulated, oxidase positive, gram positive cocci
B. The outer cell membrane mass is about one half lipo-oligosaccharide
C. Group B disease is most common in the UK

D. Group C disease incidence is about 50% of all cases
E. Treatment of choice is cefotaxime 50 mg/kg iv for 3 days

Q 55. Gabapentine:

A. is available only as an oral preparation
B. bioavailability varies directly with the dose
C. has direct γ-aminobutyric acid (GABA) agonist action
D. clearance is reduced by cimetidine
E. side effects include somnolence, dizziness and ataxia

Q 56. The following are anti-inflammatory cytokines:

A. interleukin-10
B. TNF receptors
C. interleukin-1 ra
D. platelet activating factor (PAF)
E. C5a

Q 57. Mivacurium:

A. is suitable for day case surgery
B. has a shorter onset of action as compared to vecuronium
C. has predominantly hepatic metabolites
D. clinically effective dose is 0.2 mg/kg
E. is more appropriate for use in asthmatics than vecuronium

Q 58. Paramagnetic analysers:

A. measure diamagnetic gases
B. can be used to measure nitric oxide
C. contain a powerful magnetic field
D. are very accurate but have a relatively short operating life
E. require no calibration

Q 59. Appropriate treatment for chest pain in a patient with aortic stenosis associated with sinus tachycardia and a blood pressure of 140/90 includes:

A. sublingual nitroglycerine
B. propranolol
C. diazepam

D. supplementary oxygen
E. sodium nitroprusside

Q 60. The dose of bupivacaine required for spinal anaesthesia is reduced in the pregnant patient at term because of decreased:

A. CSF volume
B. spinal cord blood flow
C. metabolism of bupivacaine
D. CSF pressure
E. turnover of CSF

Q 61. Treatment with lithium:

A. causes leukopenia
B. is associated with hypothyroidism
C. induces hyperkalaemia
D. causes an exaggerated reaction to sedative drugs
E. antagonises the action of suxamethonium

Q 62. Inorganic fluoride is a normal metabolite of:

A. halothane
B. desflurane
C. isoflurane
D. enflurane
E. cyclopropane

Q 63. Causes of increased bleeding during head and neck surgery include:

A. hypoxia
B. hypocarbia
C. respiratory obstruction
D. chronic aspirin therapy preoperatively
E. transfusion of excessive quantities of blood

Q 64. The essential diagnostic criteria for brain stem death include:

A. a serial flat EEG
B. a normal blood glucose

C. no convulsive activity
D. absent corneal reflexes
E. no reflex movement of the limbs

Q 65. The following are the effects of intermittent positive pressure ventilation:

A. reduced functional surfactants
B. increased alveolar capillary permeability
C. a reduced inflammatory response in the alveoli
D. increased mortality in critically ill patients
E. increased risk of nosicomal infection

Q 66. In a patient with established renal failure:

A. chest infection is better treated with aminoglycoside antibiotics
B. hypertension is always present
C. there is a progressive rise in CVP
D. suxamethonium is contraindicated
E. there is delayed gastric emptying time

Q 67. Helium:

A. is stored as a liquid in a brown cylinder
B. has the same viscosity as oxygen
C. supports combustion
D. reduces the work of breathing in asthma
E. produces a change in the voice

Q 68. The following are recognised features of an acute pulmonary embolism:

A. a normal chest X-ray
B. ECG signs of left ventricular strain
C. pleuritic chest pain
D. preference for sitting upright
E. raised levels of D-dimers

Q 69. In capnography the CO_2 tension can be measured using:

A. mass spectrometer
B. gas chromatography

Paper 5

Questions

C. infrared spectrometer
D. photo acoustic spectrometer
E. Raman scattering

Q 70. A 70-year-old female patient presented with dehydration after persistent vomiting for 24 h due to small bowel obstruction. She is tachycardic, hypotensive, tachypnoeic on air. The following would be present:

A. hypoxia
B. uraemia
C. hyperglycaemia
D. respiratory alkalosis
E. metabolic acidosis

Q 71. The appropriate iv treatment for ventricular arrhythmias developing during anaesthesia includes:

A. digoxin 500 μg over 30 min
B. lidocaine 50 mg over 2 min up to 200 mg over 5 min
C. calcium gluconate
D. propranolol 10 mg iv
E. amiodarone 150 mg over 10 min

Q 72. The application of a topical anaesthetic agent to the pyriform fossa produces anaesthesia to the:

A. recurrent laryngeal nerve
B. glossopharyngeal nerve
C. hypoglossal nerve
D. superior larygeal nerve
E. ansa hypoglossi

Q 73. The principles involved in intra-operative oxygen analysis include:

A. oxygen extraction
B. absorption of oxidative energy
C. paramagnetism
D. Graham's law
E. the volumetric method

Q 74. In a patient with a penetrating chest injury, hypotension and an elevated CVP the following would be appropriate:

A. increased FiO_2
B. restriction of iv fluids
C. insertion of a chest drain
D. IPPV
E. ketamine induction of anaesthesia

Q 75. Venous thromo-embolism is associated with:

A. arrhythmia
B. deceased end-tidal CO_2
C. hypotension
D. constricted peripheral circulation
E. gallop rhythm

Q 76. Polycystic renal disease:

A. can affect both the kidney and the liver
B. is a hereditary disease
C. seldom causes hypertension
D. is associated with a short life expectancy
E. is a contraindication to renal transplant

Q 77. The likely causes of the development of tachycardia and systolic hypertension in a patient with adult onset diabetes mellitus, controlled with diet and oral hypoglycaemics during enflurane anaesthesia include:

A. hyperosmolar hyperglycaemia
B. surgical stimulation
C. ketoacidosis
D. hypercarbia
E. hypokalaemia

Q 78. Concerning ECG changes during anaesthesia:

A. Preoperative calcium channel blockers prevent intra-operative ischaemic ST segment changes
B. Verapamil is the drug of choice for acute atrial fibrillation

C. Propranolol controls tachycardia associated with laryngoscopy
D. Complete heart block is best treated with epinephrine
E. Phenytoin is useful for digoxin induced arrhythmia

Q 79. Pressure gauges:

A. reduce high pressure to low pressure
B. regulate the flow of gas from a cylinder
C. are calibrated in newtons
D. form part of a device for measuring gas flow
E. utilise the Bourdon gauge principle

Q 80. The following vaporisers have a temperature-compensating device on the outlet of the vaporiser chamber:

A. EMO vaporiser
B. Fluotec Mark II
C. Miniature Oxford vaporiser
D. Dräger vapour vaporiser
E. Fluotec Mark III

Q 81. Malignant hyperthermia is characterised by:

A. rapid uptake of calcium ions by the sarcoplasmic reticulum in the presence of halothane
B. an impairment of ATPase activity in the sarcoplasmic reticulum
C. decrease in skeletal muscle pH
D. rapid catabolism of muscle glycogen
E. depletion of muscle creatinine phosphate stores

Q 82. "Off-pump" coronary by-pass (OPCAB) surgery is contraindicated:

A. in patients with calcified coronary arteries
B. in the presence of fast atrial fibrillation
C. when there is cardiomegaly
D. in the presence of poor left ventricular function
E. in the elderly (over 70 years)

Q 83. Surgical diathermy:

- **A.** uses high frequencies to reduce the chance of electrocution
- **B.** uses a damped wave for coagulation
- **C.** uses a pulsed wave for cutting
- **D.** isolating capacitor has low impedance to the frequency of 1 MHz.
- **E.** current density is high at the neutral plate

Q 84. The risk of explosion is:

- **A.** low at the stoichiometric concentration
- **B.** higher in air than oxygen alone
- **C.** higher when nitrous oxide is mixed with oxygen than with oxygen alone
- **D.** increased with pure oxygen under pressure
- **E.** less when plastic (PVC) tracheal tubes are used than with red rubber tubes

Q 85. Acute peptic ulceration:

- **A.** is common after ingestion of paracetamol
- **B.** is frequently multiple
- **C.** usually causes perforation
- **D.** sometimes occurs in the duodenum soon after severe burns
- **E.** generally responds to appropriate antibiotic treatment

Q 86. With regard to liver transplants:

- **A.** renal function should be optimised
- **B.** preoperative liver enzymes should be corrected to normal
- **C.** nitrogen balance should be controlled
- **D.** ascites should be controlled
- **E.** infusion of blood is contraindicated

Q 87. The following cranial nerves carry pre-ganglionic parasympathetic nerves:

- **A.** oculomotor nerve
- **B.** trigeminal nerve
- **C.** facial nerve
- **D.** vagus nerve
- **E.** cochlear nerve

Q 88. Causes of calcification on CXR include:

A. asbestosis
B. mitral stenosis
C. sarcoidosis
D. varicella zoster virus infection
E. rubella

Q 89. In a 20-year-old woman with pre-excitation tachycardia of Wolff-Parkinson-White (WPW) syndrome:

A. narrow complex tachycardia is usually regular
B. amiodarone is contraindicated
C. digoxin is contraindicated
D. verapamil is useful in irregular broad-complex tachycardia
E. ventricular fibrillation (VF) is always stopped by amiodarone

Q 90. Polymorpho-nuclear leukocytes in CSF may be a feature of:

A. carcinomatosis of the meninges
B. tabes dorsalis
C. acute infective polyneuritis
D. tuberculous meningitis
E. acute poliomyelitis

Table for your Answers

Question	A	B	C	D	E
1					
2					
3					
4					
5					
6					
7					
8					
9					
10					
11					
12					
13					
14					
15					
16					
17					
18					
19					
20					
21					
22					
23					
24					
25					
26					
27					
28					
29					
30					

Question	A	B	C	D	E
31					
32					
33					
34					
35					
36					
37					
38					
39					
40					
41					
42					
43					
44					
45					
46					
47					
48					
49					
50					
51					
52					
53					
54					
55					
56					
57					
58					
59					
60					

Question	A	B	C	D	E
61					
62					
63					
64					
65					
66					
67					
68					
69					
70					
71					
72					
73					
74					
75					
76					
77					
78					
79					
80					
81					
82					
83					
84					
85					
86					
87					
88					
89					
90					

Section 3 – Answers

Paper 1 Answers

A 1. **A.** true **B.** true **C.** true **D.** true **E.** false

The problems associated with laparoscopy are caused by:

- Intra-peritoneal insufflation
- Absorption of carbon dioxide
- Positioning
- The surgical procedure

Respiratory effects

These effects are due to the:

- Pneumo-peritoneum
- Use of carbon dioxide as the insufflation gas
- Position of the patient

The lung volumes are reduced, especially the functional residual capacity (FRC) due to displacement of the diaphragm cephalad, reduced chest wall dimensions and muscle tone with a reduced intrathoracic blood volume. These changes lead to atelectasis, pulmonary shunting and hypoxaemia.

Increased airway pressures may result in:

- Barotrauma and pneumothorax
- Increased physiological dead space
- Reduced lung compliance
- Hypercarbia as carbon dioxide is absorbed
- Endobronchial intubation as the carina moves cephalad

Cardiovascular effects

Secondary to pneumo-peritoneum, the effects of the GA and positioning are:

- Increased systemic vascular resistance
- Increased mean arterial pressure
- Decreased pre-load leading to reduced cardiac output
- Ischaemia due to alterations in supply and demand

- Arrhythmias – These may be ventricular due to rise in carbon dioxide tension or vagally mediated due to peritoneal traction
- Cardiac failure

Additional problems are:
- Acid aspiration and regurgitation
- Deep vein thrombosis
- Trocar injuries to bowel and bladder
- Bleeding
- Postoperative nausea and vomiting
- Venous gas embolism
- Burns and explosions

A 2. **A.** true **B.** true **C.** true **D.** true **E.** false

Bowel obstruction
The clinical features of prolonged bowel obstruction include:
- Vomiting, colicky abdominal pain, abdominal distension, absolute constipation (i.e. neither flatus nor faeces)
- Dehydration and loss of skin turgor
- Hypotension and tachycardia
- Abdominal distension and increased bowel sounds
- Empty rectum on digital examination
- Tenderness or rebound indicates peritonitis

A 3. **A.** false **B.** false **C.** true **D.** true **E.** true

Acute tubular necrosis
Acute tubular necrosis (ATN) accounts for 85% of the intrinsic causes of acute renal failure (ARF).

Causes
- 50% are due to ischaemia
- 35% are due to toxins – inflammatory mediators, aminoglycosides, paracetamol, heavy metals and myoglobin

The thick ascending limb (TAL) of the Loop of Henle is particularly predisposed to ischaemia for two reasons.
1. Although total blood flow to the kidneys is very high (25% of cardiac output) the majority is directed to the renal cortex. Medullary blood flow is limited so that the concentration gradient of osmolarity is preserved.
2. Active ion pumps in the TAL are high oxygen consumers.

The combination of poor blood supply and high oxygen demand leaves this section of the tubule very vulnerable to ischaemia.

Plasma biochemistry
- Rising urea and creatinine
- A metabolic acidosis, with or without hyperkalaemia

Urinary analysis
Loss or tubular concentrating ability in intrinsic ARF results in urine and plasma that are iso-osmolar.

Typical findings:
- Oliguria <30 ml/h of dilute urine
- Urine osmolarity <350 mosmol/l
- Urine sodium >20 mmol/l
- Urine urea <150 mmol/l
- Urine specific gravity <1,010
- Ratio of urine to plasma osmolarity <1:2
- Ratio of urine:plasma creatinine <20
- Pigmented casts in urine

A 4. **A.** false **B.** true **C.** true **D.** false **E.** false

ABO compatible platelet transfusions are desirable but not essential. Platelet concentrates contain small numbers of RBCs and leukocytes. They can be stored at 22°C to 24°C for 5 days but platelet function deteriorates after 48 h. They are administered through a special filter, do not require cross matching, contain citrate as an anticoagulant and do not result in significant release of histamine.

A 5. **A.** true **B.** true **C.** false **D.** false **E.** false

The following types of agents have been used:
- Phenothiazines – a group of anti-psychotic (neuroleptic) drugs have a limited role in the treatment of vomiting
- Butyrophenones – effective in the prevention and treatment, of postoperative nausea and vomiting
- Benzamides
- Metoclopramide used as an antiemetic and prokinetic drug
- Antagonism of peripheral D1 receptors resulting in vasoconstriction of renal and mesenteric vasculature

Paper 1 Answers

A 6. **A.** true **B.** true **C.** false **D.** false **E.** true

Vitamin B_{12} is indicated in the following conditions:

- Individuals with pernicious anaemia
- Individuals with gastro intestinal disorders
  - Sprue, coeliac disease, regional enteritis, localised inflammation of the stomach or small intestine
- Partial and total gastrectomy when the antrum and intrinsic factor is lost
- Vegetarians who do not eat meat, fish, eggs, milk or milk products

A 7. **A.** true **B.** true **C.** true **D.** true **E.** false

Causes and associations of aortic regurgitation are:

Acute regurgitation causes

- Acute rheumatic fever
- Infective endocarditis
- Dissection of the aorta
- Ruptured sinus Valsalva aneurysm
- Failure of a prosthetic valve

Chronic aortic regurgitation

- Rheumatic heart disease
- Syphilis
- Arthritides: Reiter's syndrome, ankylosing spondylitis and rheumatoid arthritis
- Severe hypertension
- Marfans' syndrome
- Bicuspid aortic valve
- Osteogenesis imperfecta

A 8. **A.** false **B.** false **C.** true **D.** true **E.** false

Fat embolism is most closely associated with fractures of the pelvis and long bones of the lower extremity. Although injury is the main triggering factor leading to fat embolism syndrome, orthopaedic procedures such as hip arthroplasty and intra-medullary nailing for lower limb fractures may lead to the release of marrow fat into the circulation.

Fat embolism may develop in any condition where there is potential for fat to be release into the circulation such as muscle injury and burns.

Of those patients who develop clinically evident fat embolism syndrome 20% show a fulminating course with mortality approaching 50%. The condition may occur at any age but it is most commonly seen in young males who are most at risk from serious trauma.

Clinical diagnosis

- P_aO_2 <8 kPa (60 mmHg)
- Petechial rash
- Unexpected neurological signs

Supportive changes

- Associated hypovolaemia and tachycardia
- Hypothermia
- Pyrexia
- Sudden reduction in haemoglobin
- Sudden onset of thrombocytopenia
- Increased erythrocyte sedimentation rate
- Fat globules in urine and sputum
- Retinal changes

A 9. **A.** true **B.** true **C.** true **D.** true **E.** true

Normal pressure is 15 to 25 mmHg. Once the eye is opened intra-ocular pressure (IOP) is equal to atmospheric pressure. IOP is increased by hypoxia, hypercarbia, coughing and vomiting.

All volatile agents cause a dose related decrease on IOP due to decreased extra-ocular muscle tone and increased aqueous humour outflow.

Etomidate and propofol reduce IOP and thiopentone reduces it but to a lesser degree. Ketamine increases IOP and causes blephorospasm and nystagmus.

All non-depolarising drugs lower IOP. Suxamethonium increases IOP possibly by contraction of the orbital smooth muscle. A peak increase occurs at about 4 min returning to normal by 6 min.

A 10. **A.** true **B.** true **C.** true **D.** false **E.** false

Surfactant is a lipid surface tension lowering agent.

Composition

- Dipalmityl phosphatidyl choline 60%
- Phosphatidyl glycine 5%

- Other phospholipids 10%
- Neutral lipoids 13%
- Proteins 8%
- Carbohydrates 2%

Synthesis

It is produced by type II alveolar epithelial cells (these are cuboid cells with large nuclei).

Functions

- It lowers the surface tension in the alveoli, so increasing the compliance of the lungs and reduces the work of breathing
- Promotes alveolar stability
- Helps to keep the alveoli dry

A **11.** **A.** true **B.** true **C.** true **D.** false **E.** true

The maxillary nerve passes through the foramen rotundum into the pterygopalatine fossa and via the fissure into the infra-temporal fossa and continues as the infra temporal nerve.

The maxillary nerve gives off numerous branches:

- Meningeal branches within the cranium (dura mater)
- Ganglionic branches within the pterygopalatine fossa (to the pterygopalatine ganglion
- Zygomatic branches within the pterygopalatine fossa divide into two branches – facial and temporal – to the cheek and temple
- Posterior superior alveolar nerve divides into branches within the pterygopalatine fossa which supply the maxillary sinus, maxillary molar teeth, cheek and gums
- Middle superior alveolar nerve – from the infra orbital nerve to the maxillary sinus and upper premolar teeth
- Anterior superior alveolar nerve from the infra orbital nerve to the maxillary sinus and canine and incisor teeth
- Intraorbital nerve divides into palpebral, nasal and superior labial branches

A **12.** **A.** false **B.** false **C.** true **D.** true **E.** true

The possible causes of renal failure during the postoperative period are:

Pre-renal

- Hypovolaemia, inadequate pre-operative correction of third spaces losses, e.g. septicaemia, pancreatitis. These cause

secretion of antidiuretic hormone (ADH), rennin and aldosterone and afferent arterial vaso-constriction
- Low cardiac output
- Hepato-renal failure associated with jaundice

Renal
- Old age
- Pre-existing renal impairment
- Renal ischaemia – thrombus or embolism
- Hypoxia
- Nephrotoxic drugs – NSAIDs, contrast media, gentamicin
- Rhabdomyolysis
- Hypercalcaemia, hyponatraemia

Post renal
- Ureteric obstruction by myoglobin, ligatures, fibrosis, tumours
- Catheter – blocked

A **13.** **A.** true **B.** true **C.** true **D.** false **E.** false

The rise in pulmonary pressures associated with venous air embolism may predispose to a right to left shunting in any condition in which a communication exists between the systemic and the pulmonary circulations. This will result in a systemic air embolism.

Such conditions are an ASD, VSD, PDA and a patent foramen ovale, which may be present in up to 35% of all individuals in autopsy studies and other complex cardiac anomalies.

A **14.** **A.** true **B.** true **C.** false **D.** false **E.** false

The differential diagnosis of bilateral lymphadenopathy includes – lymphoma, pulmonary tuberculosis, carcinoma of the bronchus and sarcoidosis (erythema nodosum).

A **15.** **A.** true **B.** false **C.** false **D.** true **E.** true

Blood gas analysers report a wide range of results, but the only parameters measured directly are:
- The partial pressure of oxygen PO_2
- The partial pressure of carbon dioxide PCO_2
- Blood pH

The haemoglobin oxygen saturation (HbO_2%) is calculated from the PO_2 using the oxygen dissociation curve and assumes a normal P50 and that there are no abnormal forms of haemoglobin present.

The actual bicarbonate, standard bicarbonate and base excess are calculated from the pH and PCO_2 using the Siggard–Anderson nomogram. This normogram is derived from a series of in vitro experiments relating pH, PCO_2 and bicarbonate.

Anaesthesia and Intensive Care Medicine December 2002; 3: 474

A **16.** **A.** false **B.** false **C.** false **D.** true **E.** false

The heart is denervated and will therefore only respond to circulating catecholamine. If there is no extra adrenaline stimulus the heart rate will be about 60 bpm. In the presence of adrenaline there will be a high resting rate, in the absence of a vagal inhibition. Typically 100 to 120 bpm. A slowing heartbeat is a sign of rejection.

The cardiovascular responses to laryngoscopy are still evident via the adrenal axis but they are often delayed.

There is no vagal tone in the transplanted heart therefore atropine is ineffective as a chronotope.

Isoprenaline is the drug of choice in a bradycardia. Anti-rejection therapy should be monitored.

BJA 1990; 67: 772–778

A **17.** **A.** false **B.** false **C.** true **D.** false **E.** true

Low molecular weight heparins are derived from the depolymerisation of heparin by either chemical or enzymatic degradation.

Compared to unfractionated heparin, low molecular weight heparins are more effective at inhibiting factor Xa and less effective at promoting the formation of the inactive "anti-thrombin – thrombin" complex.

Advantages
- Single daily dose due to a longer half-life
- Less effective on platelets
- Reduced affinity for von Willebrand factor

- Reduced risk of heparin induced thrombocytopenia
- Reduced need for monitoring coagulation

Protamine is not fully effective in reversing the effects of low molecular weight heparin.

Kinetics

- Administered subcutaneously once a day (bioavailability is 90% from the subcutaneous route)
- The half-life is 12 h, which is 2 to 4 times longer than standard heparin
- Less protein bound than standard heparin
- Renal elimination and the $t_{1/2}$ increases with renal failure

A 18. A. true **B.** false **C.** true **D.** true **E.** true

Auto PEEPi (intrinsic PEEPi) is the difference between the alveolar pressure and the airway pressure at the end of expiration. It exists when expiration continues right up to inspiration (i.e. there is no expiratory pause).

PEEPi occurs when there is:

- An obstruction to expiratory flow – asthma, chronic obstructive ariway disease (COAD)
- When the expiratory time is too short – rapid respiratory rate, prolonged inspiratory time

Newer ventilators usually have a means of checking the PEEPi level. It is important to note that the value on the pressure dial of ventilators during expiration does not reflect the level of PEEPi in the lung.

When beneficial, PEEP increases FRC by alveolar recruitment. This reduces pulmonary venous admixture and increases P_aCO_2 at any given FiO_2. However PEEP may produce unpredictable effects especially if lung compliance is dyshomogeneous, as in pneumonia or volume-controlled ventilation. PEEP will increase peak airway pressure and may cause over distension of lung units, hence:

- Barotrauma is a risk
- Compression of vessels around distended alveoli may divert blood to underventilated regions, hence:
  - Increased physiological dead space
  - Worsen the shunt fraction
  - Increased pulmonary vascular resistance (PVR)

A 19. A. false **B.** true **C.** false **D.** false **E.** true

Ecstasy (3,4 methylenedioxymethamphetamine – MDMA) is an amphetamine derivative.

MDMA causes the release of 5-HT, one of the neurotransmitters implicated in the control of mood. In primates it causes irreversible loss of serotonergic nerve fibres. 5-HT is a neurotransmitter triggering the thermoregulatory centre in the hypothalamus to increase body temperature.

Acute effects include:

- Empathy
- Heightened alertness
- Acute psychosis
- Trismus
- Tachycardia

Positive effects tend to lessen with regular use while negative effects increase.

The main problems in the management of these patients are:

Acute toxicity
Hyperthermia, muscle rigidity, obtunded consciousness and fitting.

There appears to be no relationship between effects and the dose. A syndrome similar to malignant hyperpyrexia can occur with rhabdomyolysis, DIC and MOF. Rapid cooling and the use of dantrolene have been recommended if the core temperature is >40°C.

Drinking large amounts of water at raves to prevent dehydration causes dilutional hyponatraemia and cerebral oedema.

Acute liver failure may occur due to either a reaction to ecstasy itself or a reaction to a contaminant.

Hall. Ecstasy and Anaesthesia. *BJA* 1997 [Editorial]

A 20. A. false **B.** true **C.** false **D.** true **E.** false

A 21. A. false **B.** false **C.** true **D.** true **E.** false

Nitrous oxide affects vitamin B_{12} synthesis by inhibiting the enzyme methionine synthetase. This effect is of importance if the duration of the nitrous oxide anaesthesia exceeds 8 h.

Nitrous oxide also interferes with folic acid metabolism and impairs the synthesis of DNA. Prolonged exposure may cause agranulocytosis and bone marrow aplasia. Exposure of patients to nitrous oxide for 6 h or longer may result in megaloblastic anaemia. Occupational exposure to nitrous oxide may result in a myeloneuropathy. This condition is similar to sub acute combined degeneration of the spinal cord and has been reported in some dentist and in individuals addicted to the inhalation of nitrous oxide.

A **22.** **A.** false **B.** true **C.** true **D.** false **E.** false

Inadvertent spinal tap is a well-recognised complication of epidural analgesia. The incidence is around 1% in obstetric practice. Headache occurs in around 80% typically from 2 to 24 h post puncture. The headache is thought to be due to loss of CSF via the tear resulting in traction on the intracranial contents. A reduction in CSF pressure may lead to cerebral vasodilatation and headache.

The presentation of the patient with headache, photophobia and hyperaesthesia of both lower limbs may suggest spinal cord compression by an epidural haematoma or abscess.

Epidural haematoma is very rare but classically presents with a sharp radiating back pain and a sensorimotor deficit. Early symptoms of an epidural abscess include headache and backache, which may be most severe at the epidural site. Later signs are of bladder and bowel disturbance which may occur with or without signs in the lower limbs.

Headache due to a CSF leak is not associated with neurological signs in the lower limbs, bladder or bowel function.

Once symptoms have developed, urgent decompression is required within 8 h to prevent permanent neurological damage.

A **23.** **A.** false **B.** true **C.** false **D.** false **E.** false

Performance of this block takes advantage of the tight neural bundle containing the brachial plexus in the infraclavicular area, anterior to the coracoid process before the nerve fibres enter the axilla. At the mid-point of the clavicle the plexus lies approximately 3 to 5 cm from the skin surface and is posterior and lateral to the subclavian artery.

Complications include pneumothorax, haemothorax, and chylothorax (with a left sided block).

A **24.** **A.** false **B.** true **C.** false **D.** true **E.** true

The ethical and legal dilemmas of withdrawing or withholding life saving treatment in children are discussed by Street K.

Street K. *British Journal of Intensive Care* 1999: 165–166

A **25.** **A.** true **B.** false **C.** true **D.** false **E.** false

Stimulation of the trigeminal nerve during posterior fossa surgery may cause arrhythmias, severe hypertension and bradycardia. The motor nucleus are in the pons leading to masseter contraction, the sensory nuclei are in the medulla, mid-brain and pons. Vagal stimulation may occur leading to hypotension and bradycardia.

A **26.** **A.** true **B.** true **C.** true **D.** true **E.** false

Considering that 15% of the population are said to be alcoholics and that 10% or more of hospital admissions are related to alcohol abuse, it is curious that anaesthetists do not encounter more problems with such patients.

Alcohol is a potent toxin that affects all systems.

Cardiovascular
Chronic abuse can lead to global cardiomyopathy, pulmonary hypertension, arrhythmias.

Thiamine deficiency can lead to high output cardiac failure.

Central nervous system
Chronic ingestion may cause neuropsychiatry abnormalities. Neuropathy and myopathy may occur.

GIT
Gastric hyperacidity, gastroparesis and reflux oesophageal diseases are common. Portal hypertension secondary to cirrhotic

liver disease causes oesophageal varices. Haematology anaemia nutritional deficiency and or chronic gastrointestinal blood loss.

Hepatic
The liver has a huge functional reserve and can continue to metabolise most drugs even in the presence of widespread pathological changes. Protein metabolism is decreased so levels of coagulation factors may be reduced (prolonged PT). Albumin levels are reduced (decreased binding of drugs).

Immune system
Excessive alcohol consumption is immunosuppressive.

Respiratory system
- Ciliary dysfunction
- Leukocyte inhibition
- Surfactant inhibition
- Postoperative chest infection

Metabolism
- Tendency to hypoglycaemia
- Withdraw symptoms

A **27. A.** false **B.** false **C.** false **D.** false **E.** false

The appropriate drug treatment of acute bronchoconstriction includes:
- Oxygen in as high a concentration as possible
- β-2 agonists starting with nebulised salbutamol in oxygen 2.5 to 5 mg and repeated. If there is no response or deterioration, this may be given intravenously at a dose of 3 to 20 μg/min
- Anticholinergics – Nebulised in oxygen ipratropium bromide 250 to 500 μg, synergistic with β-2 agonists
- Aminophylline – This is a controversial drug and is generally used in patients who have failed to respond to the above therapy
- Steroids – The role of steroids in the acute severe bronchoconstriction is established and they should be given early after presentation of symptoms
- Fluids and electrolytes
- Regular assessment
- Other less well established treatments include: magnesium, adrenaline, ketamine, inhalation volatile anaesthetic agents and helium

Paper 1

Answers

A 28. **A.** false **B.** false **C.** false **D.** false **E.** true

The potential complications of coeliac plexus block are:

- Injection into aorta, vena cave, left renal artery
- Intraperitoneal injection
- Retroperitoneal haematoma
- Backache
- Hypotension
- Diarrhoea
- 0.15% risk of paralysis
- 3% risk of impotence
- Acute ischaemic myelopathy

A 29. **A.** false **B.** false **C.** true **D.** true **E.** false

A 30. **A.** true **B.** true **C.** true **D.** false **E.** false

This is an intrinsic muscle disorder. There is delayed muscle relaxation due to an abnormal closure of the sodium/chloride channels following depolarisation. This causes repetitive discharge and contraction.

Clinical features

- General classic triad: frontal baldness/cataracts/mental retardation
- Skeletal muscle atrophy leading to weakness of facial, neck, respiratory and distal musculature
- Failure of muscle relaxation (myotonia) following voluntary or induced contraction (shivering, TENS, diathermy)
- Pharyngeal muscle weakness, which may lead to aspiration
- Cardiac problems – first degree heart block, mitral valve prolapse (20% of cases), cardiomyopathy
- Endocrine problems – gonadal atrophy, infertility, diabetes mellitus, hypothyroidism, adrenal insufficiency
- Respiratory system – central sleep apnoea
- Symptoms deteriorate during pregnancy (uterine atony)

A 31. **A.** true **B.** true **C.** false **D.** true **E.** false

This occurs in any condition in which communication between systemic and pulmonary circulation is present allowing a right to left shunt. ASD, VSD, PDA, tetralogy of Fallot, patent foramen ovale.

A 32. **A.** true **B.** true **C.** false **D.** true **E.** true

Hepatic encephalopathy is a metabolic disorder of the central nervous system and neuromuscular system that may complicate liver failure from any cause. It is particularly associated with advanced cirrhosis on account of the diffuse parenchymal damage and post systemic shunting.

The condition may be precipitated by:

- Diarrhoea – Hypokalaemia increases renal ammonia production. Alkalosis increases the amount of ammonia that crosses the blood brain barrier
- Constipation
- Diuretics
- Vomiting
- GIT bleeding
- Infection
- Sedatives
- Paracetamol
- High protein diet
- Metabolic disturbance, e.g. hypoglycaemia

A 33. **A.** false **B.** false **C.** true **D.** false **E.** false

If intravenous cannulation is difficult an interosseous infusion can provide emergency vascular access in children less than 6 years of age.

A rigid 18 G spinal needle within a stylet or shorter bone marrow trephine needle can be inserted into the distal femur or proximal tibia. If the tibia is chosen, a needle is inserted 2 to 3 cm below the tibial tuberosity at a 45° angle to the skin and away from the epiphyseal plate.

Once the needle is advanced through the cortex it should stand upright without support.

Proper placement is confirmed by the ability to aspirate marrow through the needle. The interosseous route is effective for:

- Fluid therapy
- Drugs epinephrine (use a higher dose than recommended for iv route)
- Induction and maintenance of anaesthesia
- Antibiotics

- Seizure control
- Inotropic support

There is a risk of osteomyelitis and compartment syndrome so it is recommended that the iv route should be established as soon as possible.

Morgan, Mikhail. *Clinical Anaesthesiology*, 2nd Edn

A **34.** **A.** false **B.** false **C.** false **D.** false **E.** true

The alveolar to arterial oxygen difference is the difference between the partial pressure of oxygen in the alveoli and the arterial partial pressure of oxygen.

The mean alveolar P_AO_2 is calculated using the alveolar air equation:

$$P_AO_2 = P_IO_2 - P_ACO_2/R + F$$

where:

- P_IO_2 is the partial pressure of inspired oxygen
- P_ACO_2 is the partial pressure of alveolar carbon dioxide
- R (the respiratory quotient) is normally between 0.7 and 0.8
- F is a correction factor

The PaO_2 is obtained from arterial blood gas analysis. The $P(A\text{-}a)O_2$ is normally 1 to 2 kPa or 5 to 10 mmHg. The difference is due to physiological shunts. It normally increases with age and inspired oxygen concentration.

A **35.** **A.** false **B.** false **C.** false **D.** true **E.** true

The effects of old age on morbidity and mortality in anaesthesia are:

Cardiovascular system

- Ischaemic heart disease
- Impaired cardiac performance
- Impaired perfusion of vital organs
- Atherosclerosis and hypertension

Respiratory system

- Increase closing capacity
- More airway collapse and greater A-a difference

- Decreased sensitivity to carbon dioxide
- Increased incidence of atelectasis, pulmonary embolism and postoperative chest infection

Nervous system

- Cerebrovascular impairment
- Hearing and sensory impairment
- Confusion

Pharmacology

- Increased sensitivity to sedatives, opioids and other drugs
- Impaired drug distribution, metabolism, elimination
- Altered plasma proteins and drug binding to proteins

Metabolism

- Slower metabolic rate
- Impaired renal blood flow and function
- Impaired fluid balance and especially dehydration
- Tendency to diabetes mellitus
- Malnourishment

Other considerations

- Physically frail with liability to damage of skin, bones, impaired temperature control
- Increased likelihood of gastro-oesophageal reflux
- Cervical spondylosis and arthritis with limitation of movement
- Thin skin

Prescribers Journal 1997; 237: 166

A 36. **A.** false **B.** false **C.** true **D.** true **E.** true

The efficacy of magnesium is now established and should be the first line therapy. The Collaborative Eclampsia Trial showed it to be clearly superior to phenytoin and diazepam.

Magnesium works by preventing cerebral vasospasm through the block of calcium influx via NMDA glutamate channels.

Magnesium sulphate is the drug of choice in eclampsia because it is more effective than diazepam and phenytoin in preventing fits and it minimises maternal mortality.

Magnesium therapy

- Dose 4 g bolus over 10 min iv followed by an infusion of 1 to 2 g/h

- Therapeutic blood levels are 2 to 3.5 mmol/l
- Treatment is continued for 24 h after the last seizure. Magnesium 1 g = 4 mmol

Magnesium in anaesthesia

- Reduces acetylcholine release
- Decreases the sensitivity of the motor end plates to acetyl choline thus increasing the sensitivity to both depolarising and non-depolarising drugs
- Placental transfer causes poor neonatal muscle tone and respiratory depression
- Reduces uterine contractility (tocolytic)

A 37. A. true **B.** false **C.** false **D.** true **E.** true

Viral properties

- Double stranded DNA virus
- Primary infection usually in first decades
- Establishes a latent infection in the dorsal root ganglion. Recurrent disease caused by a viral reaction

Disease loci

- Dorsal root ganglion especially the thoracic dermatomes
- Pain deep aching or burning
- Dysaesthesia, paraesthesia
- Allodynia
- Post herpetic neuralgia pain >1 month after eruption may persist for >3 months

A 38. A. false **B.** true **C.** true **D.** true **E.** false

Scoliosis is a lateral curvature of the spine often with a rotational element. The deformity usually arises in late childhood and may be postural or structural.

Postural scoliosis arises as a compensatory mechanism for problems outside the spine such as a shortened leg or abnormal pelvic tilt.

Structural scoliosis is a fixed deformity and is always accompanied by bony abnormalities.

Adolescent idiopathic scoliosis is the most common form, presenting in the 10–15 age group.

Operative treatment is indicated for a curvature of over 40°.

Surgery to the upper thoracic spine is achieved by a modified and extended cervical exposure, mid-thoracic spinal surgery is most easily performed via a thoracotomy. A trans-diaphragmatic approach involving detachment of the diaphragm is required for lower thoracic procedures.

The degree of risk of spinal cord damage depends on the extent of the vertebral disease and the extent of the reconstruction required.

Blood pressure control is important; balancing the need to ensure spinal cord perfusion with the desire to produce a bloodless field. Sodium nitroprusside and esmolol infusions have been widely used for this purpose.

Neurophysiological monitoring using spontaneous evoked potentials (SEPs) provides a continuous picture. The electrical stimuli are applied to the lower limbs and appropriate placed electrodes can record cortical (SCEP) or spinal (SSEP) evoked potentials.

A **39.** **A.** true **B.** false **C.** false **D.** false **E.** false

Initial treatment depends on the degree of dehydration.

For *severe dehydration* >15% loss of body weight with severe alkalaemia and impending circulatory failure.

- Correct the deficit with a bolus of 20 ml/kg crystalloid 0.9% saline or colloid

For *mild to moderate dehydration* 5 to 10% loss of body weight with moderate alkalaemia (bicarbonate 32 to 42 mmol/l)

- Give glucose saline plus 10 mmol of KCl per 100 ml at 6 to 8 ml/kg/h. Plus nasogastric losses as ml of saline

Target for fluid therapy:

- Serum chloride 106 mmol/l
- Serum sodium 135 mmol/l
- Serum bicarbonate 26 mmol/l
- Urinary chloride 20 mmol/l
- Urine output >1 ml/kg/h

Maintenance fluid therapy:

- Glucose 4% with saline 0.18% saline. Plus potassium supplements 10 mmol KCl per 500 ml bag at 4 ml/kg/h

A 40. **A.** true **B.** true **C.** true **D.** false **E.** false

The mean resting cerebral blood flow in young adults is about 50 ml/100 g brain tissue/min. There are however regional differences in blood flow with mean values for grey matter of 870 ml/100 g brain/min and white matter 20 ml/100 g brain/min.

The brain accounts for 20% of basal oxygen consumption and 25% of basal glucose consumption. Under normal circumstances this is more than adequately met by the 15% of the cardiac output that the brain receives (750 ml/min in adults).

The physiological determinates of cerebral blood flow and volume are:

- Regional metabolism – Increases in local neural activity are accompanied by increases in regional cerebral metabolic rate this is termed flow-metabolism coupling
- Cerebral perfusion pressure CPP = MAP − (ICP + CVP), where CPP = cerebral perfusion pressure; MAP = mean arterial pressure; ICP = intracranial pressure; CVP = central venous pressure at jugular bulb (usually zero)

$PaCO_2$ – partial pressure of carbon dioxide in arterial blood
$PaCO_2$ affects cerebral blood flow through vasodilatation by changing the pH of the extra cellular fluid. Cerebral blood flow varies linearly with $PaCO_2$ in the range between 3.0 and 7.0 kPa and declines at both ends of the range. A 3% change in cerebral blood flow occurs for each 0.1 kPa change on $PaCO_2$. PaO_2 has less influence on cerebral blood flow until PaO_2 is less than 8.0 kPa.

Temperature
Cerebral blood flow increases by 5 to 7% for every 1°C rise. Hypothermia decreases both CMR and CBF.

Autonomic nervous system

- Mainly affects the larger cerebral vessels
- β-1 adrenergic stimulation results in vasodilatation
- α-2 adrenergic stimulation leads to vasoconstriction

A 41. **A.** false **B.** true **C.** false **D.** true **E.** false

Acute myocardial infarction has a mortality of 25%. Over half of the deaths occur within the first hours usually associated with ventricular fibrillation.

The ECG changes

After the first few minutes:

- T waves become tall and pointed and upright
- ST segment elevation

After the first few hours:

- T waves invert
- The R wave voltage is decreased
- Q waves develop

After a few days:

- The ST segment returns to normal

After weeks:

- The T waves may return to normal
- Q waves remain

Persistent ST segment elevation may be due to:

- Acute pericarditis
- Acute cor pulmonale
- Hypokalaemia
- Ventricular aneurysm

A 42. **A.** true **B.** true **C.** false **D.** true **E.** false

Symptoms of a pneumothorax

- Shortness of breath
- Pleuritic pain

Signs of a pneumothorax

- Inspection and palpation – decreased expansion
- Percussion – increased percussion note
- Auscultation – decreased breath sounds and decreased SaO_2

Tension pneumothorax

As above plus:

- Contralateral mediastinal shift
- Cardiovascular collapse

A 43. **A.** false **B.** false **C.** true **D.** true **E.** true

The knee jerk is a monosynaptic stretch reflex. Stimulus = tap the patellar tendon stretches the quadriceps muscle. The sense organ is the muscle spindle.

Afferent fast sensory fibres – type Ia
Centrally, the nerves enter the dorsal horn of the spinal cord and synapse with the cell bodies of the motor neurones.

Efferent
α-neurones supply the muscle. Response = contraction of the quadriceps.

A 44. **A.** true **B.** true **C.** false **D.** true **E.** false

The risks are such that no child less than 60 weeks should undergo surgery unless absolutely essential. The risks are related to apnoeic spells, which may occur as late as 12 h following surgery in about 20 to 30% of healthy neonates. Prolonged observation is necessary and respiratory stimulants may be required. The risks of apnoea decrease with increasing gestational age and local anaesthetic techniques may also reduce the risk of this complication.

Other risks include bradycardias, hypothermia and hypoglycaemia. Premature babies should have their maturity assessed from 40 weeks gestation not from the time of the birth.

Crane PM. Anaesthesia for the premature born infant. *Current Anaesthesia and Critical Care* 2000; 11: 245–249

A 45. **A.** true **B.** true **C.** false **D.** true **E.** false

The pattern of spontaneous respiration has been used to indicate brainstem integrity but the improved surgical fields obtained with IPPV are striking. In the paralysed patient, proximity to the vital structures is indicated by dramatic changes in pulse, cardiac rhythm and blood pressure.

A 46. **A.** true **B.** false **C.** false **D.** false **E.** false

Tramadol is an opioid analgesic drug introduced into the UK in 1994 but used in other countries for years before.

It is a weak μ-agonist with even weaker activity at the κ and δ subtypes of opioid receptor.

It inhibits the neuronal uptake and promotes the release of both norepinephrine (noradrenaline) and 5-hydroxytryptamine.

It undergoes renal excretion and metabolism.

Half-life = 6 h.

Side effects include:

- Nausea and vomiting
- Dry mouth
- Dizziness
- Confusion
- Hallucinations
- Sweating
- Convulsions

It appears to produce minimal tolerance and dependence and relatively little respiratory depression.

BJA 1998; 81: 51–57

Anaesthesia and Intensive Care Medicine 2001; 2: 11

Paper 1 Answers

A **47.** **A.** true **B.** false **C.** true **D.** true **E.** true

NSAIDs inhibit the synthesis of renal prostaglandins that would normally vasodilate the afferent arterioles in the presence of low renal blood flow. NSAIDs may cause acute renal failure.

These drugs are contraindicated in patients with impending renal failure.

ACE inhibitors reduce the production of angiotensin-2 that normally constricts the efferent arterioles and are also contraindicated.

Aminoglycosides cause nephrotoxicity in a dose related manner, which is greater in the elderly.

A **48.** **A.** false **B.** true **C.** true **D.** true **E.** true

A **49.** **A.** false **B.** true **C.** false **D.** true **E.** true

Acute haemolytic transfusion reaction is usually due to an ABO, Lewis, Kell or Duffy incompatible transfusion. IgM complement mediated cytotoxicity or IgG mediated lysis of red cells results in liberation of anaphylotoxins, histamine and coagulation activation.

Intra-operative signs include:

- Fever
- Cyanosis
- Bronchospasm
- Pulmonary oedema
- Cardiovascular collapse and oozing

Treatment depends on support for organ failure.

A **50.** **A.** false **B.** true **C.** false **D.** true **E.** false

Myasthenia syndrome is a non-metastatic manifestation of carcinoma of the lung. Also known as Eaton Lambert syndrome (ELS). It is characterised by proximal muscle weakness that typically affects the lower extremities. It is more commonly associated with small cell lung carcinoma.

At the molecular level there is a pre-junctional defect in the quantal release of acetylcholine which may be due to antibodies directed against calcium channels. Clinically Eaton Lambert syndrome produces autonomic effects – hypotension, gastroparesis, urinary retention.

Exercise causes an improvement in the weakness. Anticholinesterases do not cause an improvement in the myasthenic syndrome but they do improve myasthenia gravis. Guanide hydrochloride and 4-aminopyridine often help by enhancing acetylcholine release by acting on calcium and potassium channels.

The response of patients with the myasthenic syndrome to neuromuscular blocking drugs is sensitive to both depolarising and non-depolarising muscle relaxants.

The EMG is characterised by no fade, decreased voltage and the response is improved by repetitive stimulation.

A **51.** **A.** true **B.** true **C.** true **D.** false **E.** true

Phaeochromocytoma is a tumour of chromaffin cells of neuroectodermal origin. 10% bilateral, 10% malignant, 10% extra-adrenal.

Secretes norepinephrine and epinephrine. Associated with neurofibromatosis, medullary thyroid carcinoma and multiple endocrine neoplasia-2 (MEN-2).

Symptoms

- Crisis (17% of cases) headache, sweating, palpitations, hypertension. Sustained in 65%, orthostatic hypotension
- Cardiac symptoms, mild hyperglycaemia, elevated haematocrit

A **52. A.** false **B.** true **C.** true **D.** false **E.** true

Haemophilia A – sex linked, recessive, inherited condition with reduced levels of factor VIII. Males are affected while females are carriers. Symptoms – spontaneous bleeding, mostly in joints developing into ankylosis and permanent joint deformities.

Coagulation tests:

- Prolonged partial thromboplastin time (APTT) the intrinsic pathway
- Normal whole blood clotting, normal bleeding time
- Diagnosis by assay of factor VIII: C assay
- Haemophiliacs treated with sterilised freeze-dried factor VIII. Those treated before this preparation are at risk from hepatitis B and C and HIV

Mild haemophiliacs may manage with an infusion of iv desmopressin.

Haemophilia B (Christmas disease) is a sex linked recessive inherited condition with reduced levels of factor IX. Coagulation test results are similar to haemophilia A with a reduced factor IX assay. Treatment is with factor IX. Desmopressin is not effective.

Deakin CD. Clinical notes for FRCA, 2nd Edn

A **53. A.** true **B.** true **C.** false **D.** true **E.** true

The effects of enflurane include:

CNS

- Anaesthesia
- Minimal analgesia
- Epileptogenic and excitatory muscular effect
- Increased cerebral blood flow and thus an increase in intracranial pressure

CVS

- Negative ionotrope
- Small decrease in systematic vascular resistance
- Mild reflex tachycardia
- Coronary vasodilatation
- Increased rate of phase 4 depolarisation
- Slight myocardial sensitisation to catecholamines

Respiratory System

- Dose dependent respiratory depression, which is predominantly a reduction in tidal volume
- Increase or decrease in respiratory rate
- Bronchodilator, non irritant, no increase in secretions

Others

- Muscle relaxants potentiated
- Blood pressure dependent decrease in splanchnic circulation
- Decreased renal blood flow and glomerular filtration rate
- Decreased uterine tone in pregnancy

A **54.** **A.** true **B.** false **C.** true **D.** false **E.** true

Atropine sulphate is a racemic mixture but only L atropine is active. Atropine combines reversibly with muscarinic cholinergic receptors and thus prevents access of acetylcholine to these sites. It is a competitive antagonist, which means that the effect of the atropine can be overcome by increasing the concentration of acetylcholine in the area of the muscarinic receptors.

Atropine does not result in cell membrane changes and associated inhibition of adenylcyclase or alterations in calcium ion permeability that would lead to a cholinergic response. It does not prevent the liberation of acetylcholine and does not react with acetylcholine.

Effects include:

CVS

- Tachycardia but may cause initial bradycardia thought to be due to a central vagal stimulation
- Cutaneous vasodilatation

CNS

- Excitement, hallucinations, hyperthermia especially in children, anti-Parkinsonism effect

RS
- Bronchodilatation and increased dead space, reduced secretions

GIT
- Reduced salivation
- Reduced motility
- Reduced secretions
- Reduced lower oesophageal sphincter tone

Others
- Mydriasis and cycloplegia
- Reduced sweating
- Reduced bladder and uterine tone

Contraindications
Beware glaucoma, hyperpyrexia in children, central anticholinergic syndrome.

A **55. A.** false **B.** true **C.** true **D.** false **E.** true

Carbon dioxide analysers are based on the principle that all molecules made up of two or more dissimilar atoms will absorb infrared light. Based on the Beer-Lambert Law.

The gas to be analysed can be sampled in two ways.

Sidestream
The gas is drawn off continuously, usually at about 100 to 150 ml/min from the breathing circuit into a detector chamber. For accuracy the tubing supplied should be used. The sampled gas should be returned to the breathing circuit to prevent a leak and waste. This allows lower flows to be used.

Advantages
- Lightweight connectors to the breathing circuit
- Multi-analysis is possible via the same tube

Disadvantages
- The lag time for the sample leaving the circuit to the monitor is longer
- Water vapour contamination if an HMEF is not used, mixing of fresh gas flow with expired gas can occur in the sample tubing

Mainstream
The gas to be analysed does not leave the patient circuit. A detector is placed in the gas flowing in the circuit. This technique can be used with a fuel cell for oxygen or an infrared radiation detector for carbon dioxide.

Advantages
- Immediate reading
- No water vapour contamination
- No gas lost from the circuit

Disadvantages
- Bulky attachment at patient end of circuit, only one gas can be measured at a time. Need a clean window to prevent erroneous readings

A **56. A.** false **B.** true **C.** false **D.** true **E.** false

The pulmonary artery capillary occlusion pressure is a reliable indication of left atrial and left ventricular end diastolic pressure. Normal occlusion pressure is 8–12 mmHg. It is measured by inflating a balloon at the distal end of a catheter, which is passed into the pulmonary artery. The catheter tip floats into a branch of the pulmonary artery where it wedges.

An increase in wedge pressure indicates either a high left ventricular pressure or a high left atrial pressure due to:
- Ventricular failure
- Fluid overload
- Cardiac tamponade
- Mitral stenosis

Capillary wedge pressure will overestimate left ventricular end diastolic pressure (LVEDP) in:
- Increased pulmonary blood flow
- Tachycardia, which limits left atrial emptying
- Placement of the pulmonary catheter in West zone I where it measures alveolar rather than pulmonary pressure
- PEEP
- Mitral valve disease, which increases left atrial, pressure

The wedge pressure will underestimate left ventricle end diastolic pressure in:
- Aortic stenosis
- Aortic regurgitation

- Ischaemic heart disease due to stiff ventricles
- Dilated cardiomyopathy (compliant ventricles)

A 57. **A.** false **B.** true **C.** true **D.** false **E.** true

The mixed venous oxygen blood reflects the amount of oxygen left after perfusion of the capillary beds in the systemic circulation. It is reduced when oxygen delivery to the tissues is inadequate for tissue needs.

Causes
- Decrease in arterial oxygen content
- Low cardiac output
- Increased oxygen consumption

A 58. **A.** true **B.** true **C.** false **D.** true **E.** true

Diamorphine is diacetylmorphine, which has no affinity for opioid receptors. It is a pro drug with active metabolites, which are responsible for its effects. It is 1.5 to 2.0 times more potent than morphine.

Kinetics
It has a high lipid and water solubility, which enables it to be administered in small volumes effectively by the subcutaneous route. 40% protein bound pKa 7.6, metabolised rapidly in the liver, plasma and central nervous system by ester hydrolysis to 6-monoacetylmorphine and morphine, which confer its analgesic and other effects. The plasma half-life of diamorphine itself is about 5 min.

Because of its potency and rapid onset of action it produces the greatest degree of euphoria of the opioids and subsequently has become a drug of addiction.

Peck TE, Williams M. *Pharmacology for Anaesthesia and Intensive care.* Greenwich Medical Media 2000

A 59. **A.** false **B.** false **C.** false **D.** true **E.** false

Mivacurium is a benzylisoquinolinium ester similar to atracurium. It is a chiral mixture of three stereospecific isomers in the following proportions:
- 36% cis-trans, 58% trans-trans, 6% cis-cis

The cis-cis isomer has about 10% of the potency of the other two isomers and is not metabolised enzymatically. The main advantage is its short duration of action being metabolised by plasma choline esterase. It is often unnecessary to use an anticholinesterase agent.

The onset can be accelerated by increasing the intubation dose such that 0.25 mg/kg has an onset of action of 2.5 min. High doses cause histamine release.

A 60. **A.** false **B.** false **C.** true **D.** true **E.** true

The components of the system should ideally include:

- Short parallel sided intravascular Teflon catheter
- Short length, narrow bore, stiff, non-compliant tubing containing heparinised saline
- Transducer diaphragm – non-compliant
- Resonance frequency $>$40 Hz. If the resonance frequency is less than 40 Hz, it falls within the range of the frequencies present in the blood pressure waveforms
- Optimal damping of 0.64 (0.6 to 0.7) of critical damping produces the fastest response without excessive oscillation

A 61. **A.** true **B.** false **C.** true **D.** true **E.** true

There are various techniques for measuring anaesthetic vapours. Infrared analysis for any molecule that is made up of two or more dissimilar atoms.

- Ultraviolet for halothane
- Interferometer
- Piezoelectric effect
- Gas chromatography
- Mass spectrometry
- Photo acoustic method
- Thermal conductivity

The molecular weight of isoflurane is 184, which is denser than nitrous oxide, which has a molecular weight of 44.

A 62. **A.** false **B.** true **C.** true **D.** false **E.** false

The Doppler effect is the change in the pitch of sound emitted from a rapidly moving vehicle as it passes the observer. Various uses are made of the Doppler effect in medicine. One application is the ultrasound blood flow detector.

In this device ultrasound waves from a vibrating crystal transmitter are beamed along an artery and the red blood cells reflect the high frequency sound waves. A receiving transducer incorporated into the pencil-like probe detects the reflected sound waves and because of the movement of the red cells these reflected sound waves have a Doppler change in frequency. This change in frequency is sensed electronically and is related to the velocity of the blood cells.

A **63.** **A.** false **B.** false **C.** true **D.** false **E.** false

Airflows to operating theatre should have the following characteristics:

- Pressure gradient about 35 Pa
- Air changes 20–40 times per hour
- Air flow 45 to 60 m^3/min
- Velocity 3 to 12 m/min
- Temperature 21–24°C
- Humidity about 50%

A **64.** **A.** false **B.** false **C.** false **D.** false **E.** true

The features of tricyclic antidepressant overdose include:

Cardiovascular

- Sinus tachycardia
- Dose related prolongation of the QT interval and widening of the QRS complex, ventricular arrhythmias when the QRS complex is longer than 0.18 s
- Right bundle branch block
- Hypotension or hypertension

Central effects

- Excitation
- Seizures
- Depression
- Mydriasis
- Hyperthermia

Anticholinergic

Treatment – Treatment includes gastric lavage followed by activated charcoal within 1 h of ingestion.

Seizures – a benzodiazepine.
Ventricular arrhythmias – phenytoin or lidocaine.

Inotropes should be avoided where possible as they may precipitate arrhythmias. Intravascular volume expansion is usually sufficient to correct the hypotension. Anticholinergic effects can be reversed by an anticholinesterases but this is not recommended as it may precipitate seizures, bradycardia and heart failure.

A **65.** **A.** true **B.** true **C.** false **D.** false **E.** false

Gas chromatography is used as a general term for the analytical procedure that separates a mixture into its component parts as the mixture passes through a column.

The system has a stationary phase and a mobile phase. The stationary phase is a column of fine silica aluminium coated with polyethylene glycol or silicone.

Through this column a flow of carrier gas is passed such as argon or helium. This is the second or liquid phase. Sample gases are then entered into the stream and the speed with which they pass through the column is determined by their differential solubility between the two phases.

As the solubility is temperate dependant the apparatus is maintained at a constant temperature.

This system is often termed as gas or liquid chromatograph. As the gases leave the column they pass through a detector which may be a:

- Flame ionisation detector for organic vapour
- Thermal conductivity detector for inorganic vapour
- Electron capture detector for a halogenated vapour

None of these detectors allows an absolute identification of the component gases and some knowledge of the substance prior or analysis is necessary. All assays need calibration with known concentrations of each particular gas.

A **66.** **A.** false **B.** false **C.** true **D.** false **E.** true

The measurement of cardiac output using thermodilution and heat as a detectable indicator in the blood has a number of advantages. Heat is rapidly dissipated into the tissues and there is no recirculation time or elevation of the indicator base line.

Using a pulmonary artery catheter a 10 ml bolus of saline, which used to be cold but is now at room temperature, is injected into the right atrium. The ensuing temperature change is recorded by a thermistor at the catheter tip located in the pulmonary artery.

A plot of temperature against time gives a wash out curve from which cardiac output can be calculated using a modification of the Stewart-Hamilton conservation of heat equation.

In current practice a microprocessor system measures the area under the curve and calculates cardiac output.

Sources of error

- Any circumstances that affect the temperature versus time graph
  - Intracardiac shunts
  - Severe tricuspid regurgitation or mitral regurgitation
- The presence of thrombus on the thermistor can delay cooling and rewarming
- The volume, temperature and rate of delivery of injectate
- Ventricular arrhythmias
- Distal migration of the catheter can lead to disproportionate blood flow with variability in the volume of cold bolus reaching the thermistor

A 67. **A.** false **B.** true **C.** true **D.** false **E.** false

The measures of dispersion (measures of variation, scatter and spread) are:

- *Sample range* – The difference between the highest and the lowest values
- *Percentile* – The level of measurement below or above which a specific proportion of the distribution falls
- *Variance and standard deviation* – These measure the spread of observations about the mean
  - Variance = sum of (individual observations − mean)^2 divided by the number of observations
  - Standard deviation = root of the variance
- *Coefficient of variation* – This is the ratio of the SD of a series of observations to the mean of the observations expressed as a percentage. Coefficient of variation = SD/mean × 100%

A 68. **A.** true **B.** true **C.** true **D.** false **E.** false

Type 2 respiratory failure (called "blue bloaters") is associated with oedema, cyanosis, hypoventilation and a reduced respiratory effort.

The patients are hypercapnoeic, giving rise to the following physical findings:
- Peripheral vasodilatation
- A pounding pulse
- A coarse flapping tremor of the out-stretched hands

More severe hypercapnoea leads to confusion, drowsiness and coma with papilloedema.

A 69. **A.** true **B.** true **C.** true **D.** true **E.** false

An elevated pulmonary artery pressure know as pulmonary hypertension can be caused by:
- Chronic lung disease
- Increased pulmonary blood flow because of the left to right shunt through a VSD, ASD and PDA
- Left ventricular failure
- Mitral valve disease
- Left atrial tumour or thrombus
- Pulmonary veno-occlusive disease
- Pulmonary thromboembolic disease

A 70. **A.** false **B.** true **C.** true **D.** false **E.** false

If found on preoperative examination complete heart block (even if not sustained) should be treated by temporary or permanent transvenous pacing.

The heart rate and cardiac output in complete heart block may increase in response to β stimulation, but electrical pacing should be started as soon as possible.

A 71. **A.** true **B.** true **C.** false **D.** true **E.** false

The carotid sheath contains:
- Internal carotid artery
- Internal jugular vein
- Vagus nerve and the cervical sympathetic chain in its posterior wall

A 72. **A.** true **B.** false **C.** false **D.** false **E.** false

Convulsions may occur with:

- Tricyclic antidepressant poisoning
- Antihistamines
- Phenothiazines
- Penicillins
- Any general anaesthetic agent

Diazepam 10 mg is the treatment of choice followed by phenytoin 1 g bolus iv over 4 h and 100 mg every 8 h.

A 73. **A.** true **B.** false **C.** true **D.** true **E.** true

A meta-analysis found the advantages of regional anaesthesia compared to general anaesthesia were:

- 1 month mortality 6.4% vs 9.4%
- Risk of DVT 30.2% vs 46%
- Perioperative confusion 12% vs 22.6%
- Hypoxia 35% vs 48%
- Myocardial infarction 0.9% vs 1.8%

The advantages of a general anaesthetic are less hypotension and a shorter operating time.

The technique for airway management and ventilation had no impact on the outcome measures.

There was no difference in the incidence of pneumonia, urinary retention and PONV or blood transfusion requirement between regional and general anaesthesia.

Wu CL, Fleisher LA. *Outcomes of research in regional anaesthesia and analgesia. Anaesthesia and Analgesia* 2000; 91: 1232–1242

A 74. **A.** false **B.** true **C.** true **D.** true **E.** false

Factors which affect the rate of diffusion across the cell membrane:

- The concentration gradient: Fick's law states that the rate of diffusion of a substance across unit area is proportional to the concentration gradient
- The molecular weight: Graham's law states that the rate of diffusion of a gas is inversely proportional to the square root of its molecular weight
- Increases with surface area
- Increases with lipid solubility
- Decreases with electrical charge of particle

A 75. **A.** false **B.** false **C.** false **D.** false **E.** true

Prothrombin time (PT) tests the extrinsic pathway.

The PT is measured by adding animal tissue thromboplastin and calcium to the patient's plasma.

Normal value = 12–14 s.

Prolonged PT in factor VIII deficiency, vitamin K deficiency, liver disease, and oral anticoagulant therapy and DIC.

A 76. **A.** false **B.** true **C.** true **D.** true **E.** true

Fallot's tetralogy is the most common cyanotic congenital heart disease in children who survive beyond the neonatal period.

It consists of the following features:

- VSD
- Right ventricular outflow obstruction
- Overriding aorta positioning of the aorta above the VSD
- Right ventricular hypertrophy

This combination of lesions leads to a high right ventricular pressure and a right to left shunt of blood through the VSD. Thus the patient is centrally cyanosed.

Presentation
Cyanosis, dyspnoea, worsening with exercise, fatigue, hypoxic episodes (Fallot's spells), deep cyanosis with syncope on exertion. Squatting is common to increase the systemic vascular resistance and hence increase pulmonary flow and decrease the venous return of desaturated blood from the lower limbs.

An ejection systolic murmur is present over the pulmonary area. S2 is not split. Finger clubbing and polycythaemia may be present by one year. CXR shows oligaemic lung fields and a boot shaped heart.

Treatment
Blalock shunt is performed as a palliative procedure. This is an anastomosis between a subclavian artery and the pulmonary artery. Complete surgical correction within the first 12 months is more common. Fallot's spells may need to be treated with β-blockers and diamorphine.

A **77.** **A.** true **B.** false **C.** false **D.** false **E.** false

Suxamethonium is contraindicated in:

- Patients with a history of malignant hyperpyrexia
- Anaphylaxis to suxamethonium
- Myopathies – Duchenne's and Myotonia dystrophia

Suxamethonium is also relatively contraindicated in certain conditions.

Suxamethonium increases the serum potassium by 0.2 to 0.4 mmol/l due to the fasciculations. In conditions where there is a proliferation of extra-junctional receptors the release of potassium is increased.

- Burns – the potassium may rise greatly for 6 h to 2 years after the burn
- Massive trauma
- Severe intra-abdominal infection
- Neurological diseases – spinal cord trauma causing recent paralysis. Suxamethonium can be given immediately after the injury but should be avoided from day 10 to day 100 after the injury
- Encephalitis
- Stroke
- Guillain-Barré syndrome
- Ruptured cerebral aneurysm
- Polyneuropathies
- Tetanus

A **78.** **A.** true **B.** false **C.** false **D.** false **E.** true

The immediate management of hyperthermia due to exercise includes the following.

General measures to cool the body:

- Decrease ambient temperature
  - expose patient
  - cold air fans
  - application of cold water
  - ice packs to extremities
  - cold iv fluids

Treatment of complications:

- Rhabdomyolisis – mannitol and renal failure
- Dantrolene for severe cases

General ITU measures.

A **79.** **A.** false **B.** false **C.** false **D.** false **E.** true

Continuous positive airway pressure (CPAP) is an elevation of the base line pressure throughout the respiratory cycle during spontaneous respiration. It can be applied using a facemask, tracheal tube or laryngeal mask and by a ventilator or pressure generating device. The aim is to prevent or reverse airway closure, thus maintaining or increasing FRC and therefore oxygenation. Increasing FRC may place the patient's lungs on a more favourable point on the compliance curve and thus minimise the work of breathing. CPAP is maintained at a pre-set level during inspiration and expiration.

During ventilatory CPAP inspiratory flow is made available in proportion to the patient's inspiratory effort but only to maintain the required CPAP level. If the demand valve is slow to respond or the patient has an excessive respiratory drive, flow delivery may be inadequate initially leading to a drop in the CPAP level and increased respiratory work. For breathing circuits sufficient flow must be provided throughout the respiratory cycle so that the patient's demands are always met. CPAP reduces the work of inspiration and expiration is largely passive.

A **80.** **A.** true **B.** false **C.** false **D.** true **E.** false

During a dive, the ambient pressure causes nitrogen to dissolve into the tissues. On ascent the decrease in pressure causes the nitrogen that has been dissolved in the body tissues to come out of solution. If ascent is too rapid the partial pressure of nitrogen in the tissues will rise above tissue hydrostatic pressure and gas bubbles form.

Symptoms range from pains in the tissues around joints (the classical bends) to neurological impairment such as visual disturbances, convulsions, paresis and loss of consciousness.

Nitrogen bubbles may also migrate from the tissues into the venous systems to cause a venous gas embolism.

A 81. **A.** true **B.** true **C.** true **D.** true **E.** false

Diabetic coma is usually seen in patients with insulin dependent diabetes mellitus (IDDM) and evolves over a period of one or two days. It is caused by a lack of insulin combined with an increase in glucagon, catecholamine and cortical stimulate lipolysis, free fatty acid production and ketogenesis.

Accumulation of keto-acids (β-hydroxybutyrate, acetoacetic acid and acetone) results in a metabolic acidosis. Increased gluconeogenesis and glycolysis result in hyperglycaemia which is not taken up peripherally because of the lack of insulin. The renal threshold for glucose is exceeded and glucosuria and ketonuria result in the loss of large amounts of water and electrolytes – hypovolaemia follows.

Precipitating factors include:
- Sepsis
- Surgery
- Ischemia and myocardial infarction
- Non-compliance with insulin and diet

Recognition:
- Reduced conscious level
- Ketone smell on breath
- Advanced dehydration
- Acidosis with increasing anion gap

A 82. **A.** true **B.** false **C.** false **D.** false **E.** false

Isoprenaline is a synthetic catecholamine with non-selective β-adrenoceptor action. It is predominantly a chronotrope but also has some inotropic action. As the tachycardia is achieved at the expense of increased myocardial oxygen consumption. Propranolol is a non-selective β-blocker without intrinsic sympathomimetic activity.

Atropine may cause an initial bradycardia following a small intravenous dose but the main action is a tachycardia.

Diazoxide is a vasodilator chemically related to the thiazide diuretics. It causes an increase in heart rate and cardiac output.

Trimetaphan is a competitive antagonist to nicotinic ganglionic receptors. It causes a compensatory increase in heart rate (its short action is due to being metabolised by pseudo cholinesterase).

Nifedipine is a calcium channel blocker causing a reflex increased in heart rate and contractility.

A **83. A.** false **B.** true **C.** false **D.** false **E.** true

Ankle reflex
The loss of the ankle reflex is a sign of a disorder of the lower motor neurone. The lower motor neurone is the motor pathway from the anterior horn cell (or cranial nerve nucleus) via a peripheral nerve to the motor end plate.

Causes of lower motor neuron lesions:
- Anterior horn cell – poliomyelitis, motor neurone disease
- Spinal root – cervical and lumber root lesions, neuralgic amyotrophy
- Peripheral or cranial nerve – nerve trauma, nerve compression, polyneuropathy

In multiple sclerosis there is an upper motor neurone lesion with sensory loss.

A **84. A.** true **B.** true **C.** true **D.** false **E.** false

α-adrenergic antagonists (α-blockers) prevent the actions of sympathomimetic agents on α-adrenoreceptors. Certain α-blockers (phentolamine and phenoxybenzamine) are non-specific and inhibit both α-1 and α-2 receptors while others selectively inhibit α-1 receptors (prazosin) or α-2 receptors (yohimbine).

Effects include:

Cardiovascular
- α-1 blockade results in vasodilatation and hypotension, which may be orthostatic
- α-2 blockade facilities norepinephrine release leading to tachycardia and arise in cardiac output
- Increased blood flow to skin, viscera and mucosa leading to nasal congestion

CNS
- Marked sedation
- Meiosis

Others
- Impotence and contact dermatitis

A 85. **A.** true **B.** true **C.** true **D.** true **E.** true

Dextrans are polysaccharides derived from bacterial action on sucrose.

There are three types classified according to molecular weight (40, 70 and 100 kDa).

Side effects
- Anaphylactic reactions – urticaria, hypotension, bronchospasm
- Interference with cross matching
- Coagulopathy resulting in increased bleeding time occurs due to an impaired polymerisation and reduced platelet function

A 86. **A.** true **B.** true **C.** false **D.** true **E.** false

Aortic stenosis may be associated with:
- Calcified congenital bicuspid value
- Rheumatic heart disease
- Degenerative disease

Symptoms
- Angina
- Dyspnoea
- Effort syncope – occurs only with severe stenosis

Signs
- Slow rising pulse
- A non-displaced apex beat
- A harsh ejection systolic murmur in the aortic area radiating to the carotids

Investigations
CXR is often normal. ECG – left atrial and left ventricular hypertrophy, light bundle branch block (LBBB).

Diagnosis can be confirmed by echocardiography and/or Doppler cardiography.

Valve replacement is required if symptomatic and/or the pressure gradient across the valve is more than 50 mmHg.

A 87. **A.** true **B.** false **C.** false **D.** true **E.** true

Several drugs have been used to lessen the pressor response to intubation.

Opioids

- Fentanyl 3–5 μg/kg iv
- Alfentanyl 20 μg/kg iv
- Remifentanil 1 μg/kg immediately prior to induction

Lidocaine

- 1.5 mg/kg iv

β-blockers

- Esmolol 2–5 mg/kg iv

α and β-blockers

- Labetolol 1 mg/kg iv

Others

- Magnesium sulphate and GTN

A 88. **A.** true **B.** true **C.** true **D.** false **E.** true

A pleural effusion needs to be more than 500 ml to cause much more than blunting of the costo-phrenic angle. On an erect film it produces a characteristic shadow with a curved upper edge rising into the axilla.

A 89. **A.** true **B.** true **C.** false **D.** false **E.** false

Cauda equina syndrome (CES) is a collection of signs and symptoms resulting from compression or ischaemia of the bundle of nerve roots emerging from the end of the spinal cord below the first lumbar vertebra. The classical syndrome is characterised by severe low back pain with bilateral sciatica associated with saddle anaesthesia, urinary retention and bowel dysfunction.

Causes

- Injury, herniated intervertebral disc
- Secondary to surgery, spinal or epidural anaesthesia, spinal manipulation

- Tumours, infection, vascular problems, spina bifida, spinal stenosis, later stages of ankylosing spondylitis

Red flags

Features of serious back disease:

- Severe back pain with bilateral or unilateral sciatica occurring for the first time under the age of 20 or over the age of 65 years
- Past history of cancer
- Bladder or bowel disturbance
- Anaesthesia or paraesthesia in the peri-anal region or buttocks
- Lower limb weakness
- Gait disturbances
- Sexual dysfunction

A 90. **A.** true **B.** true **C.** false **D.** false **E.** false

Cardioversion is an effective treatment for some re-entrant tachyarrhythmias, which may produce haemodynamic instability, and myocardial ischaemia and which do not respond to other measures.

Indications

- Atrial fibrillation
- Arial flutter
- Supraventricular tachycardia
- Ventricular tachycardia

The ECG monitoring lead chosen should demonstrate a clear R wave in order to synchronise the discharge away from the T wave and thus reduce the risk of developing ventricular fibrillation. If the arrhythmia does not convert after the first 50 J discharge, further shocks are given using an increased energy discharge up to 200 J.

Despite the use of a synchronised discharge ventricular fibrillation may be produced in the presence of:

- Hypokalaemia
- Ischaemia
- Digitalis intoxication
- QT prolongation cause by quinine, TCA and hyperalimentation

There is a risk of embolic phenomena in patient with:

- Mitral stenosis and atrial fibrillation of recent onset
- A history of embolic phenomena
- Prosthetic valve
- Congestive heart failure

Patients with these conditions should receive prophylactic anticoagulation.

Answers

Question	A	B	C	D	E
1	T	T	T	T	F
2	T	T	T	T	F
3	F	F	T	T	T
4	F	T	T	F	F
5	T	T	F	F	F
6	T	T	F	F	T
7	T	T	T	T	F
8	F	F	T	T	F
9	T	T	T	T	T
10	T	T	T	F	F
11	T	T	T	F	T
12	F	F	T	T	T
13	T	T	T	F	F
14	T	T	F	F	F
15	T	F	F	T	T
16	F	F	F	T	F
17	F	F	T	F	T
18	T	F	T	T	T
19	F	T	F	F	T
20	F	T	F	T	F
21	F	F	T	T	F
22	F	T	T	F	F
23	F	T	F	F	F
24	F	T	F	T	T
25	T	F	T	F	F
26	T	T	T	T	F
27	F	F	F	F	F
28	F	F	F	F	T
29	F	F	T	T	F
30	T	T	T	F	F

Question	A	B	C	D	E
31	T	T	F	T	F
32	T	T	F	T	T
33	F	F	T	F	F
34	F	F	F	F	T
35	F	F	F	T	T
36	F	F	T	T	T
37	T	F	F	T	T
38	F	T	T	T	F
39	T	F	F	F	F
40	T	T	T	F	F
41	F	T	F	T	F
42	T	T	F	T	F
43	F	F	T	T	T
44	T	T	F	T	F
45	T	T	F	T	F
46	T	F	F	F	F
47	T	F	T	T	T
48	F	T	T	T	T
49	F	T	F	T	T
50	T	T	F	T	F
51	T	T	T	F	T
52	F	T	T	F	T
53	T	T	F	T	T
54	T	F	T	F	T
55	F	T	T	F	T
56	F	T	F	T	F
57	F	T	T	F	T
58	T	T	F	T	T
59	F	F	F	T	F
60	F	F	T	T	T

Question	A	B	C	D	E
61	T	F	T	T	T
62	F	T	T	F	F
63	F	F	T	F	F
64	F	F	F	F	T
65	T	T	F	F	F
66	F	F	T	F	T
67	F	T	T	F	F
68	T	T	T	F	F
69	T	T	T	T	F
70	F	T	T	F	F
71	T	T	F	T	F
72	T	F	F	F	F
73	T	F	T	T	T
74	F	T	T	T	F
75	F	F	F	F	T
76	F	T	T	T	T
77	T	F	F	F	F
78	T	F	F	F	T
79	F	F	F	F	T
80	T	F	F	T	F
81	T	T	T	T	F
82	T	F	F	F	F
83	F	T	F	F	T
84	T	T	T	F	F
85	T	T	T	T	T
86	T	T	F	T	F
87	T	F	F	T	T
88	T	T	T	F	T
89	T	T	F	F	F
90	T	T	F	F	F

Paper 2 Answers

A 1. **A.** true **B.** true **C.** true **D.** false **E.** false

The differential diagnosis of intra-operative bronchospasm or wheezing include:

- Mechanical obstruction in the tube – kinking – secretions – over inflation of the cuff
- Inadequate depth of anaesthesia – active expiratory efforts – decreased functional residual capacity (FRC)
- Endobronchial intubation (usually with an oxygen saturation of 85 to 91%)
- Pulmonary aspiration
- Pulmonary oedema
- Pulmonary embolism
- Pneumothorax
- Acute asthmatic attack
- Anaphylaxis

A 2. **A.** false **B.** false **C.** false **D.** true **E.** false

The treatment for Parkinson's disease is aimed at restoring the dopaminergic/cholinergic balance. The levodopa increases brain levels of dopamine (dopamine itself does not cross the blood-brain barrier), by the conversion of levodopa to dopamine outside the CNS with the resultant side effects which are prevented by the current administration of carbidopa or benserazide. These inhibit dopa carboxylase peripherally, but do not themselves cross into the brain.

(Phenothiazines and butarylphenones) Droperidol antagonises central dopamine (D2) receptors at the CTZ so it should not be used.

A 3. **A.** true **B.** false **C.** false **D.** false **E.** false

In one-lung anaesthesia, the inhibitory factors to pulmonary vasoconstriction include:

- Extremes of pulmonary artery pressure
- Hypocapnia

- Low mixed venous oxygen tension
- Vasodilator therapy
- Pulmonary infection
- Possibly volatile anaesthetics

A 4. **A.** true **B.** false **C.** false **D.** false **E.** true

A 5. **A.** true **B.** false **C.** true **D.** true **E.** true

The causes of pancreatitis are:

Acute

- Gallstones, Alcohol, Infection – mumps, coxasackie B, Pancreatic tumours
- Drugs – Azathioprine, Oestrogens, Corticosteroids
- Iatrogenic – Post ERCP, post cardiac surgery
- Trauma, hyperlipidaemias, idiopathic

Chronic

- Alcoholism accounts for >80% of cases
- Idiopathic, Tropical – malnutrition, hereditary, trauma hypercalacaemia

A 6. **A.** false **B.** true **C.** false **D.** true **E.** true

Bleeding into the subarachnoid space may occur as a result of:

- Ruptured intracranial aneurysm
- Traumatic brain injury
- Ruptured arterio-venous malformation
- Idiopathic

Classically, SAH presents with:

- Sudden onset of severe headache
- Nausea and vomiting
- Meningism

Risk factors are:

- Age – most frequently between 40 and 60 years
- Hypertension
- Smoking (10-fold increase of bleeding)
- Contraceptive pill
- Cocaine abuse
- Positive family history

- Associated with Marfan's syndrome, polycystic kidneys, neurofibromatosis, and Ehlers-Damlos syndrome

Diagnosis
Non-contrast computer tomographic (CT) scan of the head demonstrates blood in the subarachnoid space in 90–95% of patients scanned within 24 h on the onset of headache. Lumbar puncture in the VCT scan is normal. Four vessel bilateral carotid and vertebral digital subtraction angiography will locate the aneurysm(s).

Management centres on the preventable morbidity and mortality from: bleeding, hydrocephalus, cerebral artery venospasm and medical complications.

Vasospasm affects 67% of patients following SAH. It is symptomatic in 32%. Typically, it presents around day 3, peaks around day 7 and resolves by day 14.

A **7.** **A.** false **B.** true **C.** false **D.** false **E.** true

Myotonica Congenita (Thompson's disease) is an autosomal dominant condition. There is an isolated myotonia, usually mild, which occurs in childhood and persists throughout life. The myotonia is accentuated by rest and cold. Diffuse muscle hypertrophy occurs and the patient appears to have well-developed muscles.

A **8.** **A.** true **B.** true **C.** false **D.** false **E.** false

Lower oesophageal sphincter tine is increased by:
- Metoclopramide
- Domperidone
- Cisapride
- Prochlorpromazine
- Neostigmine
- Pancuronium

A **9.** **A.** false **B.** false **C.** true **D.** true **E.** true

The patients most at risk for postoperative nausea and vomiting (PONV) are:

Patient factors
- Age – young; Sex – female gender
- Phase of menstrual cycle

- Motion sickness
- Smoking, obesity, anxiety, previous history of PONV, early mobilisation, eating and drinking

Surgical factors
- Nature of the operation
- Length of the operation
- ENT
- Gynaecological procedures
- Laparoscopic operations

Anaesthetic factors
- The anaesthetist, premeditation, anaesthetic agents – etomidate, N_2O, opioids, antibiotics
- Spinal or regional, peri-operative hydration
- Postoperative pain, hypotension

Efferent and afferent nerves
- Sympathetic and parasympathetic
  - Vagus (mainly)
  - Small contribution from sympathetic

Pharmacological interventions
- Phenothiazines – prochlorperazine, chlorpromazine
- Butyrophenones – droperidol
- Anticholinergics – hyoscine, atropine, cyclizine
- Antihistamines – cyclizine
- Dopamine antagonists – metoclopramide, domperidone
- 5-HT_3 receptor antagonists – ondansetron, granisetron

Others: Neurokinin receptor antagonists – cannabis.

A **10.** **A.** true **B.** true **C.** true **D.** false **E.** false

A **11.** **A.** true **B.** false **C.** true **D.** true **E.** false

High-risk groups for latex allergy include:
- Confirmed latex allergy – confirmed by skin prick or radioallergosorbet
- History of atopy and multiple allergies – may show cross reactivity with some foods (kiwi fruits)
- History of skin sensitivity to latex products such as rubber gloves
- Repeated exposure to latex products – health care workers, patients undergoing repeated catheterisation, multiple operations

Paper 2 Answers

A 12. **A.** false **B.** true **C.** true **D.** false **E.** true

Angiotensin-converting enzyme (ACE) inhibitors block the action of the carboxypeptidase ACE in the lung. This converts the inactive angiotensin I to the active octapeptide angiotensin II.

Angiotensin II causes profound vasoconstriction and causes release of aldosterone resulting in sodium and water conservation.

Effects of ACE inhibitors

CVS

Significant reduction in systemic vascular resistance results in a fall in blood pressure. Heart rate is usually unaffected but may increase. Baroreceptor reflexes are also unaffected.

Respiratory system

- Persistent dry cough – may be due to increased levels of bradykinin

Renal

- Increased renal blood flow – natriuresis

Metabolic

- Elevated renin level
- Hyperkalaemia, raised urea and creatinine especially in those with even mildly impaired renal function

Others

- Angio-oedema
- Agranulocytosis
- Thrombocytopenia
- Loss of taste
- Rash
- Pruritus

A 13. **A.** true **B.** true **C.** true **D.** false **E.** true

Blood stained sputum varies from small streaks of blood as in chronic bronchitis to massive fatal bleeding.

Causes

- Acute infection, particularly exacerbations of chronic bronchitis and emphysema (this is the commonest cause)
- Pulmonary infarction
- Bronchogenic carcinoma

- Tuberculosis
- Lobar pneumonia
- Pulmonary oedema with frothy sputum
- Bronchiectasis with infection

Uncommon causes
- Idiopathic pulmonary haemosiderosis
- Good Pasteur's syndrome
- Microscopic polyarteritis
- Trauma
- Blood diseases with disordered clotting
- Benign tumours
- Mitral stenosis

A **14.** **A.** false **B.** true **C.** false **D.** false **E.** true

The possible complications of deep cervical plexus block are:
- Intravascular injection into the vertebral artery causes immediate seizures or loss of consciousness
- Subarachnoid injection and total spinal
- Phrenic nerve palsy in 60% of cases
- Haematomas, hoarseness of the voice, dysphagia, stellate ganglion block – Horner's syndrome

A **15.** **A.** true **B.** true **C.** true **D.** false **E.** false

The lateral popliteal nerve (common peroneal nerve) derived form the sciatic nerve in the lower third of the thigh. It runs in the lateral part of the popliteal fossa before winding around the neck of the fibula. It then divides deep to peroneus longus into two branches:
1. Superficial peroneal nerve
2. Deep peroneal nerve

Block or damage to the nerve causes loss of foot eversion and foot dorsifexion. Plantar flexion of the foot is a function of the tibial nerve, which is the other terminal branch of the sciatic nerve. Note that S1 and S2 supply the ankle reflex.

A **16.** **A.** false **B.** false **C.** true **D.** false **E.** false

The treatment protocol for anaphylaxis is as follows:
- Stop administering the suspected agent
- Maintain the airway and give 100% oxygen

- Lay the patient flat with the feet elevated
- Adrenaline 10 μg/kg (0.5–1.0 mg) 1 in 1,000 contains 1 mg in 1 ml
- iv crystalloid

A **17.** **A.** false **B.** false **C.** false **D.** false **E.** false

The palate repair tends to lift the palate towards the roof of the nasopharynx, narrowing the airway. This may be worsened by spasm of the levator palatini. The obstruction may be overcome by inserting a nasopharyngeal airway (usually a shortened tracheal tube one size less than that used for oral intubation). Ideally the surgeon should insert this before removing the gag if the repair is tight. The nasopharyngeal airway must be kept patent post-operatively by gentle suction. The baby should be nursed on a high dependency unit.

A **18.** **A.** true **B.** true **C.** false **D.** true **E.** false

The deep peroneal nerve innervates muscle and bone underlying the dorsum and metatarsal pharyngeal joints of the second, third and fourth toes. Cutaneous innervation is limited to the adjacent sides of the great and second toes. Four branches of the tibial nerve (roots L4, 5 and S1, 2, 3) supply the skin and superficial tissues of the sole of the foot.

A **19.** **A.** true **B.** false **C.** true **D.** false **E.** false

Chronic myeloid leukaemia (CML) is a disease of middle age. The majority of patients present with tiredness, weight loss and sweating. Splenomegaly is found in 90% of cases. About 90% of cases of CML have the Philadelphia chromosome (Ph).

Symptoms
These are usually of insidious onset anaemia, sweating at night, fever, weight loss and abdominal discomfort due to splenic enlargement.

Signs
- Anaemia, splenomegaly
- Blood count
- Hb low or normal, WCC raised, platelet low normal or raised – bone marrow aspirate shows a hypercellular marrow with an increase in myeloid precursors

- Cytogenic analysis – the Ph chromosome is an abnormal chromosome 22, which forms a translocation with chromosome 9. The karyotype produced is called t(9;22)(q34;q11). Philadelphia chromosome is also found in acute lymphoblastic leukaemia.

A 20. **A.** true **B.** false **C.** true **D.** true **E.** true

The commonest cause of hyperadrenocorticism is an excess of adrenocorticotrophic hormone (ACTH), produced by tumours of the pituitary. ACTH or corticosteroid secretion from tumours of lung, pancreas, carcinoid and adrenal gland are uncommon.

Clinical presentation

- Obesity
- Osteoporosis leading to pathological fracture and spinal deformity
- Skin bruising and peripheral muscle wasting
- Psychosis
- Glucose intolerance in 60%
- Hypertension in 85% with hypernatraemia, hypokalaemic alkalosis
- Sleep apnoea
- More prone to secondary infection and thromboembolic disease

Management

- Check and treat CVS function, electrolytes and fasting blood glucose
- Care with positioning and muscle relaxants
- Steroid supplement should be limited to day of surgery in minor cases and only on subsequent days for major surgery and complications

A 21. **A.** true **B.** true **C.** true **D.** true **E.** true

Obstructive sleep apnoea affects 1 to 4% of the middle aged male population. It is a term applied when the degree of obstruction and sleep disturbance leads to daytime sleepiness.

Airway narrowing without obstruction leads to snoring. Total obstruction for more that 20 s is obstructive sleep apnoea. The morbidity, due to recurrent night time hypoxic episodes includes hypertension, myocardial ischaemia, heart failure and stroke.

Treatment is by nasal CPAP. The implications for anaesthesia are a potentially difficult airway and postoperative hypoxia. All sedative drugs can precipitate airway obstruction postoperatively.

A 22. **A.** true **B.** true **C.** true **D.** false **E.** true

Human albumin solution is prepared by fractionation of multiple units of plasma giving 96% albumin and 4% globulin. Each 20 g of albumin requires 20,000 blood donations, pasteurisation at 60°C for 10 h to kill all micro-organisms including viruses.

A 23. **A.** true **B.** false **C.** false **D.** false **E.** false

There are two general classifications of nerve injuries.

Seddon's classification describes three groups:
- Neuropraxia
- Axontemesis
- Neurotemesis

Sunderland's classification:
- Depends on which connective tissue components are disrupted
- Describes 5 types of injury

1. Neuropraxia
Sunderland type 1
- Functional loss – focal conduction block
- Pathological basis – local myelin injury, primary affects larger fibres, axon continuity, and no Wallerian degeneration

Recovery occurs in weeks depending on nerve length.

2. Axontemesis
(a) Sunderland type 2
- Functional loss – loss of nerve conduction at site of injury and distally
- Pathological basis – disruption of axonal continuity with Wallerian degeneration

Good prognosis for recovery since original end organs can be reached.

(b) Sunderland type 3
- Functional loss – loss of nerve conduction at injury site and distally

- Pathological basis – loss of axonal continuity endoneurial tubes and perineurium. Epineurium preserved

Poor prognosis. Surgery may be required.

(c) Sunderland type 4

- Functional loss – loss of nerve conduction at site of injury and distally
- Pathological loss – loss of axonal continuity and endoneurial tubes. Epineurium remains intact

Poor prognosis. Surgery necessary.

3. Neurotemesis

Sunderland type 5

- Functional loss – loss of nerve conduction at site of injury and distally
- Pathological loss – severance of entire nerve

A **24.** **A.** true **B.** true **C.** false **D.** false **E.** false

Pulmonary oxygen toxicity is related to the level and duration of raised oxygen tension. It may occur when concentrations over 60% are inhaled for prolonged periods at atmospheric pressure perhaps due to inactivation of surfactant and damage to pulmonary epithelium.

A **25.** **A.** false **B.** false **C.** false **D.** true **E.** false

The anaesthetic problems with sickle cell disease include:

- Avoidance of precipitating factors of a sickle crisis
- Difficult iv access
- Receiving long-term opioid pain relief with possible opioid tolerance
- Anaemia and high cardiac output failure
- Infection – salmonella
- Psychiatric problems coping with pain crisis and limited life expectancy
- Intra operative thrombo-embolic crises
- Acute chest syndrome
- Renal impairment
- Pulmonary hypertension
- Precipitants of a sickle cell crisis
- Dehydration, hypoxia, cold, alcohol, stress, infection, menstruation, vascular stasis, acidosis

Management principles

- Oxygen
- Crystalloid for intravascular volume
- Prevention of venous stasis and DVT prophylaxis
- Normothermia
- Transfusion to maintain oxygen carrying capacity
  - in the homozygote HbA concentrations should be >40% with a total Hb >10 g/dl
  - exchange transfusion should achieve up to 12 g/dl
- Transfusion is used for those undergoing operations and in a life-threatening crisis

A 26. **A.** false **B.** true **C.** true **D.** true **E.** true

Ankylosing spondylitis is characterised by inflammatory back pain and sacroilitis starting between the ages of 15 and 40 years. It is common, affecting about 1% of males, but with a variable severity and progression. It is much less common in women. Over 90% of patients have the HLA-B27 antigen.

Clinically it is characterised by a high ESR, fever, weight loss and anaemia. It causes progressive fibrosis, ossification and ankylosis of the sacroiliac joints and spine. 50% have an extra-articular involvement.

Anaesthetic problems include: difficult intubation as a result of limited cervical spinal movement and ankylosis of the tempero-mandibular joint with limited mouth opening in >10% of patients. Cricoarytenoid arthritis presents as dyspnoea and hoarseness. Cardiovascular complications include aortic incompetence, mitral valve disease and conduction defects. The thoracic spinal involvement limits chest expansion and is associated with pulmonary fibrosis.

A 27. **A.** true **B.** false **C.** true **D.** true **E.** false

This is a normal finding in 5% of elderly adults. It is associated with:

- Congenital heart disease – ASD, Fallot's teratology, pulmonary fibrosis, VSD
- Respiratory disease – cor pulmonale and pulmonary embolism
- Cardiac disease – acute myocardial infarction, cardiomyopathy and fibrosis in the conducting system
- Others – hyperkalaemia and antiarrhythmic drugs

A 28. **A.** true **B.** true **C.** true **D.** false **E.** false

For brain blood flow see PAPER 1, **Q** 40.

A 29. **A.** true **B.** true **C.** true **D.** true **E.** false

Passive hyperventilation causes a fall in $PaCO_2$ and (H^+), often with a small reduction in bicarbonate concentration if hyperventilation persists. Some degree of renal compensation may occur producing a metabolic acidosis, although this is unusual.

A 30. **A.** false **B.** true **C.** false **D.** true **E.** true

The ability to provide a continuous, accurate, beat to beat reproduction of the arterial waveform depends on a structured pressure transducer. The components of the system should include:

- A short, parallel-sided Teflon or polyurethane 20 G cannula inserted into one of the peripheral arteries
- A catheter – short length, narrow bore. Stiff, non-compliant tubing containing heparinised saline
- A flush system to prevent occlusion of the cannula with clots by flushing with saline at a rate of 1–4 ml/h
- A pressure transducer – a strain gauge of an electrically conductive elastic material that responds reversible to deformation by a change in its electrical resistance which can be converted into an output signal using a Wheatstone bridge, or a plate which moves as one side of a capacitor

A 31. **A.** true **B.** false **C.** true **D.** false **E.** true

A thermistor bead is made from a small bead of metallic oxide. Unlike normal metals, the resistance falls exponentially with temperature. They may be made exceedingly small and introduced almost anywhere. They have a rapid thermal equilibration and a narrow reference range so different thermistors are therefore required for different scales. Accuracy is improved by incorporation into a Wheatstone bridge. Calibration may be changed by exposure to severe temperatures (e.g. sterilisation).

A 32. **A.** true **B.** false **C.** true **D.** true **E.** true

Cushing's syndrome is caused by an excess of cortisol from steroid therapy, adrenal hyperplasia, adrenal carcinoma or ectopic ACTH. Cushing's disease is due to an ACTH secreting pituitary tumour.

Symptoms and signs

- Moon face
- Buffalo hump
- Thin skin
- Hirsuitism
- Easy bruising
- Hypertension (60%)
- Diabetes (10%)
- Osteoporosis (50%)
- Pancreatitis (2%)
- Muscle weakness
- Poor wound healing
- Perioperative problems
- Hypertension, congestive cardiac failure, hyperglycaemia

Careful positioning is required due to osteoporosis and fragile skin.

A 33. **A.** true **B.** false **C.** true **D.** true **E.** true

Oxygenated blood from the placenta passes through the single umbilical vein and enters the inferior vena cava, about 50% by-passing the liver via the ductus venosus. Most of the blood is diverted through the foramen ovale into the left atrium, passing to the brain via the carotid arteries.

Deoxygenated blood from the brain enters the right atrium via the superior vena cava and passes through the tricuspid valve to the right ventricle. Because the resistance of the pulmonary vessels within the collapsed lungs is high, the blood passes from the pulmonary artery trunk through the ductus arteriosus to enter the aortic arch down stream of the origin of the carotid arteries. Thus relatively oxygen rich blood is delivered to the brain. The rest of the body is perfused with less well-oxygenated blood. Deoxygenated blood reaches the placenta via the two umbilical arteries, which arise from the internal iliac arteries. They receive about 60% of the cardiac output.

Approximate blood gases values

Umbilical vein

- PO_2 – 4 kPa
- PCO_2 – 6 kPa
- pH – 7.2

Umbilical artery

- PO_2 – 2 kPa
- PCO_2 – 7 kPa

A 34. **A.** false **B.** false **C.** true **D.** false **E.** true

A Valsalva manoeuvre is a forced expiration against a closed glottis. It provides a good demonstration of autonomic reflex control of heart rate and blood pressure in response to a rise in intrathoracic pressure.

The normal person maintains their mean blood pressure by increasing heart rate and peripheral vascular resistance.

On release of the pressure there is a transient hypotension and bradycardia.

The Valsalva response is absent or abnormal in autonomic dysfunction as in diabetic autonomic neuropathy and sympathectomy by surgery or drugs.

A 35. **A.** true **B.** true **C.** false **D.** false **E.** true

Causes of difficult intubation include:

Congenital

- Pierre Robin syndrome, Cystic hygroma, Treacher-Collins syndrome, Achondroplasia, Marfan's syndrome

Anatomical

- Excessive weight, short muscular neck with a full set of teeth, protruding incisors, long high arched palate with a long narrow mouth, receding mandible, large swelling in the neck, mouth or upper chest, decreased distance between the occiput and the C1 spinous process

Acquired conditions

- Acute swelling due to bleeding or trauma, restricted jaw opening due to: trismus from infection, fibrosis after surgery or radiotherapy, rheumatoid arthritis or osteoarthritis of the tempero-mandibular joint

- Mandibular fracture
- Restricted neck movement
- Ankylosing spondylitis
- Cervical spine arthritis
- Neck instability
- Cervical spine injury, rheumatoid arthritis, Down's syndrome, tumours of larynx, pharynx or tongue

Charcot Marie Tooth disease is peroneal atrophy – distal limb weakness and wasting.

A **36.** **A.** false **B.** false **C.** true **D.** true **E.** true

The nitrogen balance is the difference between the amount of nitrogen ingested (as amino acids or proteins) and the amount of nitrogen excreted (mainly as urinary urea). It is usually measured in 24 h periods.

Negative balance occurs when losses exceed intake as in:

- Catabolism
- Starvation
- Adrenal cortical steroid therapy

Positive balance occurs when intake exceeds losses as in:

- Recovery from severe illness
- Growth
- Convalescence

A **37.** **A.** true **B.** true **C.** false **D.** true **E.** true

Thrombocytopenia can be caused by:

- Impaired production
- Bone marrow infiltration by leukaemia, myelofibrosis
- Drugs, radiation, megaloblastic anaemia, a plastic anaemia
- Immune destruction
- Idiopathic (ITP), SLE, heparin induced, HIV
- Peripheral consumption
- DIC, microangiopathic processes – haemolytic uraemic syndrome, thrombocytopenic purpura
- Platelet pooling – splenomegaly

A **38.** **A.** false **B.** false **C.** true **D.** true **E.** true

The hypokalaemia in patients suffering from major trauma may result from:

- Haemolysis, shifting of potassium to outside the cells, e.g. acidosis
- Decreased excretion, e.g. acute renal failure
- Rhabdomyolysis

A 39. **A.** true **B.** true **C.** true **D.** true **E.** true

Fluoroquinolones are a new group of quinolones. They are chemical modifications to the basic nalidixic acid structure. They include ciprofloxacin, ofloxacin, sparfloxacin and norfloxacin.

These agents are highly active against most common gram-negative bacteria and bowel pathogens. Activity against *Streptococcus pneumoniae* is only modest. Quinolones have no activity against anaerobic organisms or enterococci.

Fluoroquinolones are well absorbed by the gut. Absorption is best in the fasting state and is reduced when they are taken with preparations containing magnesium, aluminium, zinc or iron salts.

A 40. **A.** true **B.** true **C.** true **D.** false **E.** false

Rapid shallow breathing occurs with both hypoxaemia and hypercapnoea. It is characterised by increasing both the tidal volume and the respiratory rate.

A 41. **A.** true **B.** false **C.** false **D.** false **E.** true

In a patient with a flail chest being ventilated and losing 1.5 l/min, the ventilator adjustments should include increasing the fresh gas flow by 1.5 l/min and reducing peak inspiratory flow rate.

A 42. **A.** true **B.** true **C.** false **D.** false **E.** true

Pulmonary vascular resistance is influenced by the following factors:

- Autonomic innervation – vasomotor tone is minimal in the normal resting state and pulmonary vessels are maximally dilated. The autonomic system exerts a relatively weak influence on pulmonary vascular resistance. Increased sympathetic tone gives rise to vasoconstriction

- Nitric oxide (NO) is an important mediator of pulmonary vascular tone, causing vasodilatation
- Prostaglandin (PGI2) is an arachidonate, which is a potent vasodilator
- Endothelins are potent vasoconstrictors
- Vascular transmural pressure – the thinner vessel walls make them more prone to collapse when alveolar pressure exceeds intravascular pressure
- Positive pressure ventilation – high positive alveolar pressure can cause an increase in pulmonary vascular resistance
- Lung volume – pulmonary vascular resistance is least at FRC. As the lung increases in volume the vessels become narrowed and elongated. As volume decreases the vessels become tortuous
- Lung disease – both acute and chronic lung disease can result in significant increases in pulmonary vascular resistance
- Hypoxic vasoconstriction is a powerful physiological reflex, which diverts blood away from hypoxic areas of the lung

A **43.** **A.** false **B.** false **C.** true **D.** true **E.** true

During pregnancy, the plasma concentration of albumin is reduced to 34–39 g/l, but globulin and fibrinogen levels are increased. Overall the total plasma protein concentration falls to 65–70 g/l. These reductions in plasma proteins are associated with the following changes.

Total colloid osmotic pressure in reduced by 5 mmHg.

Drug binding capacity is reduced with consequent changes in pharmacokinetics and dynamics.

Plasma concentrations of pseudocholinesterase is reduced by 20–25% at term.

Erythrocyte sedimentation rate (ESR) and blood viscosity are increased.

A **44.** **A.** false **B.** false **C.** true **D.** false **E.** false

The supraclavicular approach to the brachial plexus can be an interscalene block. This approach anaesthetises the three trunks of the plexus which lie above the first rib.

As the lower trunk may lie under the subclavian artery, the medial antebrachial and ulnar nerves are the most likely to be missed.

A 45. **A.** true **B.** false **C.** false **D.** true **E.** true

The features of ABO incompatibility are:

- Rapid onset of fever
- Back pain
- Skin rash
- Hypotension
- Dyspnoea
- DIC renal failure may occur
- Hypotension and increased oozing of blood from wounds may be the only indications of incompatible transfusion in an anaesthetised patient

A 46. **A.** true **B.** false **C.** false **D.** true **E.** true

Nitric oxide is produced by a variety of cell types and is an important molecular messenger with many physiological roles. It is synthesised from L-arginine by a family of enzymes (the NO synthases).

These enzymes are of three main types:

1. Endothelial synthase (ENOS)
2. Neuronal synthase (NNOS)
3. Macrophage synthase (MNOS)

The endothelial and neuronal synthases are normal constituents in endothelium, platelets, myocardium and skeletal muscles.

They are calcium calmodulin dependent and cause continuous NO synthesis in small amounts in response to cellular activation.

The biological action of NO is short lived as it has a 10^5 fold higher affinity for haemoglobin than oxygen (half-life = 5–7 s).

NO reacts with both oxy and deoxy Hb to form methaemoglobin (metHb) and nitrosylHB respectively.

The macrophage NO synthase (pathological) is an inducible enzyme. It is not calcium dependent.

It is produced by endothelium, myocytes and macrophages in response top cytokines, microbes and endotoxins.

It causes the release of large amounts of NO, which is cytotoxic in high concentration.

The therapeutic dose of NO in ARDS is 5 to 80 ppm.

Paper 2

Answers

A 47. **A.** true **B.** false **C.** true **D.** true **E.** false

The clinical features of small bowel obstruction are:

- Vomiting, colicky abdominal pain, abdominal distension, absolute constipation (i.e. neither faeces nor flatus)
- Dehydration and loss of skin turgor
- Hypotension and tachycardia
- Increased bowel sounds
- Empty rectum on digital examination
- Tenderness or rebound indicates peritonitis

A 48. **A.** true **B.** false **C.** true **D.** true **E.** true

Normal mixed venous oxygen saturation is approximately 75%. It reflects the amount of oxygen left after perfusion of the capillary beds in the systemic circulation.

It is decreased when oxygen delivery to the tissues is inadequate for tissue needs (supply exceeds demand) in:

- Reduced arterial oxygen content
- Reduced cardiac output
- Increase in oxygen uptake (rise in VO_2)

The most common causes are:

- Low cardiac output
- Anaemia

Mixed venous oxygen saturation (SVO_2) is increased with:

- Sepsis
- Cyanide poisoning
- Left to right shunt
- Hypothermia
- A wedged PA flotation catheter

Bersten AD, Soni N. *Oh's Intensive Care Manual*, 5th Edn. Butterworth Heinemann, 2003

A 49. **A.** false **B.** true **C.** false **D.** true **E.** true

The base deficit is the amount of acid or base in mmols required to restore one litre of blood to normal pH at a PCO_2 of 5.3 kPa at body temperature.

By convention, its value is negative in acidosis and positive in alkalosis.

It may be read from the Siggaard-Anderson normogram.
It is useful as an indication of the severity of the metabolic component of acid-base disturbance and in calculating the appropriate dose of acid or base required to treat.

A 50. **A.** true **B.** true **C.** true **D.** true **E.** true

The triggering agents for malignant hyperthermia (MH) are:

- Inhalational anaesthetic agents
  - Halothane
  - Enflurane
  - Isoflurane
  - Sevoflurane
  - Desflurane
- Suxamethonium

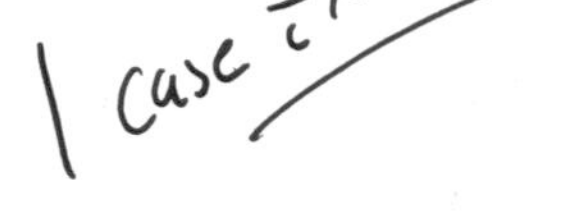

A 51. **A.** true **B.** false **C.** false **D.** true **E.** true

With laser surgery, there is a risk of fire and explosion in the airway. There is a risk of igniting the tracheal tube and burning the cornea.

The trachea should be shielded from the laser by wrapping with aluminium foil or using a tube which is resistant to burning such as one impregnated with carbon or made from a flexible metal. A double cuff can be used so that if one is burnt the other one still makes seal. The cuffs should be filled with water to absorb heat.

Oxygen and nitrous oxide support combustion. The risk of fire is reduced by keeping the $F_IO_2 < 40\%$, by adding helium and by using the laser for as short a period as possible. Swabs soaked in water are used to protect the surrounding tissues.

All theatre staff should wear protective goggles.

Plastic tracheal tubes are particularly at risk from burning with a thick black smoke.

A 52. **A.** false **B.** false **C.** false **D.** true **E.** true

Contact of blood with plastic surfaces and filters activates the clotting cascade. Anticoagulation is therefore required to prevent thrombus deposition in the circuit.

Agents
- Heparin 5–10 units/kg/h
  - Systemic, local or in priming fluid
  - The aim is to keep the APTR at 2.0 to 2.5
- LMWH
- Epoprosterol (prostacyclin) 2.5–10 ng/kg/min may be used as an alternative to prevent heparin-induced thrombocytopenia.

A 53. **A.** false **B.** false **C.** true **D.** false **E.** true

Phenytoin

Unfortunately there is no ideal drug. There have been many attempts to determine the optimum treatment regime for status epilepticus. A recent 5-year randomised multicentre study compared four options for the initial intravenous therapy. In this study:
- Lorazepam 0.1 mg/kg was effective as an initial therapy in 65% of patients
- Phenobarbitone 15 mg/kg was effective as an initial therapy in 58%
- Diazepam 0.15 mg/kg followed by phenytoin 18 mg/kg was effective as an initial therapy in 56%
- Phenytoin 18 mg/kg was effective as an initial therapy in 44%

The initial dose of phenytoin in status epilepticus is 20 mg/kg given as 50 mg/min with further doses of 5–10 mg/kg up to a total of 30 mg/kg.

A 54. **A.** false **B.** true **C.** false **D.** false **E.** true

Hyaline membrane disease is the most common cause of RDS and respiratory failure during the first few days of life.

It is commonly due to prematurity. Before 34–36 weeks gestation there is both insufficient alveolar development and a lack of surfactant.

Predisposing factors:
- Prematurity
- Male gender
- Caucasian
- Delivered by caesarean section
- Child of a diabetic mother
- Multiple pregnancy

Most cases of RDS resolve within 4–5 days with endogenous surfactant production. If supplemental oxygen is insufficient the addition of CPAP is very useful.

A 55. **A.** true **B.** true **C.** false **D.** true **E.** false

Subtotal thyroidectomy is a surgical treatment for hyperthyroidism. The postoperative complications include:

- Bleeding is the commonest serious event leading to stridor and possible life threatening airway obstruction
- Unilateral recurrent laryngeal nerve palsy leading to hoarseness
- Tracheal oedema
- Pneumothorax
- Thyroid crisis
- Hypoparathyroidism causes hypocalcaemia and tetany may occur after several hours or days

A 56. **A.** true **B.** true **C.** true **D.** false **E.** true

The normal total bilirubin concentration (conjugated and unconjugated) is less than 1.5 mg/dl (<25 μmol/l) and reflects the balance between production and biliary excretion. Jaundice is usually clinically obvious when total bilirubin exceeds 3 mg/ml.

A predominantly conjugated hyperbilirubinaemia (>50%) is associated with increased urinary urobilinogen and may reflect:

- Hepatocellular dysfunction
- Intrahepatic cholestasis
- Extrahepatic biliary obstruction

Hyperbilirubinaemia that is chiefly unconjugated may be seen with:

- Haemolysis
- Congenital or acquired defects in bilirubin conjugation

A 57. **A.** true **B.** true **C.** true **D.** true **E.** false

The oral contraceptive pill leads to an increases in fibrinogen, a hypercoagulable state and an increased incidence of venous thrombo-embolism.

Prostate resection may lead to the release of pro-coagulant material into the circulation and result in a consumptive coagulopathy.

A 58. **A.** true **B.** false **C.** false **D.** false **E.** false

Xenon is a colourless, odourless noble gas, which has been proposed as a replacement for nitrous oxide. It is the only inert gas with anaesthetic properties at ambient pressure, having:

- MAC of 71%
- the lowest blood/gas partition coefficient of any anaesthetic gas (0.11)

Advantages

- Rapid induction and recovery
- Analgesia
- Not harmful to the environment
- Cardiovascular stability
- Useful identification of mechanisms of anaesthesia
- Probably not a cause of malignant hyperpyrexia

Disadvantages

- Avoid in patients with raises intracranial pressure until its safety is proven. It has a variable effect on cerebral blood flow
- Very expensive
- Postoperative nausea and vomiting could be a problem

Prepared from air where it is present in concentrations of 0.000009%.

A 59. **A.** true **B.** true **C.** false **D.** false **E.** false

In a patient who has sustained a head injury the priorities are to avoid hypoxia, hypercarbia and hypotension to prevent secondary brain damage.

General measures include:

Airway
Unstable cervical spinal injury should be assumed until excluded. The airway should be secured if there is any doubt that there may be airway compromise of GCS <8 after resuscitation.

Breathing
All head injury patients requiring intubation will need ventilation support. Ventilation should be monitored by arterial blood gases. The aim is PaO_2 >13 kPa, $PaCO_2$ 4–4.5 kPa. Hyperventilation may induce a fall in cardiac output and local vasoconstriction, which will result in a reduced cerebral blood flow.

Circulation

- Insert a large bore (14 G) iv cannula
- Ensure normovolaemia
- Maintain MAP >90 mmHg, CPP >70 mmHg
- With iv fluids and vasoconstrictors and inotropes

Disability

- Rapid assessment of GCS should be undertaken before and after induction
- Papillary signs
- Posturing
- Cushing response (increased blood pressure with bradycardia)
- *Exposure* to identify other injuries
- *Ensure* adequate levels of sedation analgesia
- *Control of seizures* and paralysis if needed
- *Identify head injures* that require neurosurgery to decompress a blood clot or elevate a depressed fracture
- *CT scan* is needed to diagnose haematomas and depressed skull fractures that may benefit from surgical intervention
- *Correct abnormal saline* and water concentrations to achieve homeostasis
- *Keep blood glucose* in range of 6–10 mmol/l
- *Prevent pyrexia*
- The patient should be admitted to an intensive care unit for further monitoring and management

A 60. **A.** true **B.** false **C.** true **D.** false **E.** false

Patients with aortic stenosis should not exert themselves and in particular they should not take part in strenuous physical exercise. Angina is best treated by supplementary oxygen and β-blockade. Vasodilators such as glyceryl trinitrate or isosorbide dinitrate may aggravate exertional syncope.

Antibiotic prophylaxis against infective endocarditis should be given.

A 61. **A.** false **B.** false **C.** false **D.** true **E.** true

In 1956, Leyland Clarke developed the polographic oxygen electrode for measuring the partial pressure of oxygen. Prior to this the partial pressure of oxygen had not been measured. Then the Severinghaus carbon dioxide electrode was developed in 1958, which revolutionised arterial blood gas analysis.

PO_2 may also be measured using the:
- Fuel cell
- Paramagnetic analysis
- The optode
- Mass spectrometry

Oxygen is a paramagnetic gas and does not absorb infrared radiation.

A **62.** **A.** true **B.** false **C.** true **D.** false **E.** false

A **63.** **A.** true **B.** true **C.** true **D.** false **E.** true

Portal hypertension occurs as a result of increased resistance to portal venous blood flow. It is said to be pathological when >12 mmHg although pressures upto 50 mmHg may occur. The spleen enlarges and anastomoses may open between the portal and systemic circulation. Some collaterals, which most commonly occur at the oesophago-gastric junction, umbilicus and rectum, may become very large with a risk of bleeding.

Causes
- Cirrhosis – due to many causes. In UK the single most common cause of cirrhosis is secondary to alcohol
- Portal vein thrombosis
- Budd-Chiari syndrome – thrombosis or obstruction of portal vein due to tumour, haematological disease or the oral contraceptive pill
- Tumours
- Cholangiocarcinoma
- Hepatocellular carcinoma
- Constrictive pericarditis
- Right heart failure

A **64.** **A.** true **B.** false **C.** true **D.** true **E.** false

Humidity can be measured by:

Hair hygrometer
This is based on the principle that hair elongates as the humidity rises, very simple and cheap. Only really accurate over the range 30–90%.

Wet and dry bulb hygrometer
The temperature of the bulb is reduced due to evaporation. The lower the humidity the greater the temperature difference. Tables are used to relate the room temperature to % humidity.

Regnault's hygrometer
This uses the principle that condensation occurs when the air is fully saturated at a given temperature. This is the Dew Point. Air is blown through a silver tube containing ether. This reduces the temperature of the tube by evaporation. When the temperature falls to the point that condensation occurs on the outside of the tube the Dew Point has been reached. From the room temperature and the Dew Point relative and absolute humidity are obtained.

Relative humidity = saturation vapour pressure at the Dew Point/saturation vapour pressure at ambient temperature.

Other methods
- Electrical transducer both resistance and capacitance
- Mass spectrometry
- Ultraviolet absorption spectroscopy

A **65.** **A.** false **B.** false **C.** true **D.** false **E.** true

Rheumatoid arthritis is common, chronic, systemic condition producing:
- A systemic inflammatory polyarthritis
- Extra-articular involvement
- Progressive joint damage causing severe disability

Pathogenesis
The cause of rheumatoid arthritis is unknown. Toxic substances produced by the inflammatory reaction in the synovium are thought to lead to the destruction of cartilage. The characteristic features of progressive rheumatoid arthritis are:

Cardiovascular manifestations
- Pericardial effusion or tamponade
- Constrictive pericarditis
- Diffuse myocarditis
- Myocardial granuloma leading to conduction defects
- Valvular heart disease – the mitral valve is affected more than the other valves

Acanthosis Nigricans
This is a localised hyperpigmentation seen in middle aged patients with visceral malignancies.

Multiple mononeuropathies (mononeuritis multiplex)
This occurs as a result of vasculitis associated with rheumatoid arthritis.

A **66.** **A.** false **B.** true **C.** false **D.** true **E.** true

Peribulbar block was first described by Davies and Mandel in 1986. The aim is to keep the needle always at a tangent to the globe, advancing the needle tip no further than the equator of the globe, outside the muscular cone. The technique uses larger doses of local anaesthetic and a longer time for onset. Use a 25 mm 25 G blunt, short bevel needle.

Technique
Insert the needle at the fornix of the conjunctiva, at the junction of the lateral third and medial two thirds. The needle is directed towards the floor of the orbit and 4 to 10 ml of local anaesthetic are injected.

It may be necessary to supplement the first injection by inserting a needle medial to the caruncular lacrimalis to a depth of 20 mm and inject 2 to 5 ml of local anaesthetic. The eyeball should be gently compressed for 10 min after the injection to aid the spread of local anaesthetic. A facial nerve block is not required.

A **67.** **A.** true **B.** true **C.** false **D.** false **E.** true

Complex regional pain syndrome (CRPS) – Type I called reflex sympathetic dystrophy and Type II called causalgia in the past – is a disorder of unknown aetiology. It presents in a limb following:

- A minor injury
- An obvious nerve injury
- Surgery
- Associated medical condition such as stroke, myocardial infarction, neurological trauma

It is a syndrome of:

- A diffuse burning limb pain
- Sensory changes include allodynia, hypoaesthesia, and hyperaesthesia

- Autonomic disturbances
  - Swelling, abnormal reduced skin circulation, abnormal sweating
  - Trophic changes – Shiny skin, coarse hair, thickened, brittle nails, muscle wasting, osteoporosis
- Motor changes are not necessary for a diagnosis but the following may occur
  - Weakness, tremor, stiffness

If untreated, the clinical picture usually goes through three stages:

- *First stage* (days and months after injury) – pain, oedema, warm, red, dry skin
- *Dystrophic stage* (3–6 months after the onset of symptoms) – pain, muscle wasting, pale, cyanotic skin
- *Atrophic stage* (6–8 months after the onset of symptoms) – pain may diminish, cool limb, contractures, severe osteoporosis

There are two types of CRPS with defined diagnostic criteria:

- *Type I* – formerly known as reflex sympathetic dystrophy or Sudeck's atrophy
- *Type II* – formerly know as causalgia. Type II is associated with an obvious nerve injury where as Type 1 is not associated with such a nerve injury

A 68. A. true **B.** false **C.** true **D.** true **E.** true

See PAPER 2, Q 9.

A 69. A. true **B.** false **C.** true **D.** true **E.** false

Induction agents

- Propofol – large volume of distribution 750 l, little change in pharmacokinetics
- Barbiturates – decreased dose requirement of thiopentone due to decreased protein binding and increased blood-brain barrier permeability
- Etomidate – decreased dose requirement due to reduced protein binding
- Ketamine – increases renal blood flow through altered autoregulation but reduces urine output

Inhalational agents
Renal toxicity of fluoride ions (enflurane and methoxyflurane) causes a high urine out flow renal failure. The minimum toxic level is 5 mmol/l.

Opioids
The effect of morphine is prolonged due to reduced renal excretion and accumulation and also reduced excretion of metabolites (M6G). Pethidine causes excitation due to accumulation of renal excreted metabolites norpethidine.

Muscle relaxants
Suxamethonium action is prolonged due to low plasma cholinesterase depleted by dialysis.

Clearance of non-depolarising drugs depends on the degree of renal excretion:

- >70% pancuronium, piperauronium, gallamine
- <25% vecuronium, atracurium, mivacurium
- Vecuronium accumulates with repeated doses
- Mivacuronium and doxacurium actions are prolonged due to reduced renal excretion
- Atracurium little change in pharmacokinetics
- Rocuronium mostly excreted through the liver

A **70. A.** false **B.** false **C.** false **D.** false **E.** true

Leukaemia is rare, with an annual overall incidence of 5 per 100,000. Both subtypes of acute leukaemia can occur in all age groups but acute lymphocytic leukaemia (ALL) is predominantly a disease of childhood, whereas acute myeloid leukaemia (AML) is most frequent in older adults.

Clinical features
The symptoms of acute leukaemia are a consequence of bone marrow failure:

- Symptoms of anaemia tiredness, weakness, shortness of breath on exertion
- Repeated infection – sore throat, pneumonia
- Bruising and/or bleeding
- Occasional lymphadenopathy, lymph node enlargement and or symptoms related to enlargement of liver or spleen

Signs (there may be few or no signs)

- Signs of anaemia
- Bruises, petechial haemorrhages, purpura, fundal haemorrhages
- Signs of infection
- Sometimes peripheral lymphadenopathy and/or hepato-splenomegaly

Blood count

- Low Hb
- WCC usually raised but can be decreased or normal
- Platelets usually reduced

Peripheral blood film
Shows characteristic leukaemia blast cells.

Bone marrow aspirate
Usually shows increased cellularity with a high percentage of abnormal lymphoid blast cells.

A 71. **A.** true **B.** true **C.** false **D.** false **E.** false

A 72. **A.** false **B.** true **C.** true **D.** true **E.** true

The alveolar – arterial oxygen pressure difference is the difference between the partial pressure of oxygen in the alveoli and the arterial partial pressure of oxygen $P(A\text{-}a)O_2$. The $P(A\text{-}a)O_2$ is normally 10–20 mmHg or 1–2 kPa. This difference is due to physiological shunts such as through bronchial and coronary circulation.

Ventilation to blood flow mismatches
In the absence of disease the difference increases with age and with increasing F_IO_2. In disease the increase in the difference is due to:

- Anatomical shunts
- Ventilation to perfusion mismatches
  - Ventilation abnormalities – reduced FRC, pneumonia, anaesthesia
  - Perfusion abnormalities – hypovolaemia, low cardiac output
- Diffusion defects
- ARDS

A **73.** **A.** true **B.** true **C.** false **D.** false **E.** false

The beneficial effects of positive end-expiratory pressure (PEEP) include:

- An increase in FRC by recruitment of partially closed alveoli
- Improvement in lung compliance
- Correction of ventilation to perfusion abnormalities

The overall result is an improvement in oxygenation.

The adverse effects include:

- Barotrauma from too high pressure, which may lead to pneumothorax, pneumo-mediastinum, pneumo-pericardium and subcutaneous emphysema
- Rise in intrathoracic pressure and may compromise venous return if the patient is hypovolaemic, leading to reduced cardiac output. This usually occurs with PEEP in excess of 10 cmH_2O
- Rises in central venous pressure, which may lead to a rise in intracranial pressure
- Decreased renal blood flow
- Decreases hepatic blood flow

A **74.** **A.** false **B.** false **C.** true **D.** false **E.** true

Adreno-cortical insufficiency can be due to:

- Auto-immune disease
- Tuberculosis
- Adrenal infiltration by myeloid disease, tumour or leukaemia
- Pituitary failure
- Surgical adrenalectomy
- Hypophysectomy

The symptoms and signs of insufficiency are not usually present until at least 80 to 90% of the glands have become destroyed or non-functioning. Any stress can precipitate an adrenal crisis in patients with adrenal suppression, but most commonly these are surgical, trauma or sepsis. A crisis can occur when long-term corticosteroid therapy is discontinued.

Presentation
Unexplained hypotension, hyperkalaemia, hyponatraemia, hypoglycaemia and reduced levels of consciousness.

Emergency treatment
Cardiovascular support – Fluid replacement of extracellular deficit with 0.9% normal saline (large volumes may be required). Urine output and CVP guide treatment. Vasopressors may be required.

Steroid therapy
Consider mineralocorticoid and glucocorticoid. Hydrocortisone 100 mg iv followed by 100–200mg daily in divided doses.

Use dextrose as necessary and treat the cause of the crisis.

A 75. **A.** false **B.** false **C.** false **D.** false **E.** false

The reaction of a single muscle fibre to a stimulus follows an all or none pattern. In contrast the response of the whole of the muscle depends on the number of muscle fibres activated.

If a nerve is stimulated with sufficient intensity all the muscle fibres supplied by that nerve will respond with a maximum response. After the administration of a neuromuscular blocking drug the response of the muscle decreases in proportion to the number of fibres blocked. The reduction in response during constant stimulation reflects the degree of neuromuscular blockade. Therefore, the stimulus must be maximal throughout the period of monitoring.

Supramaximal stimulus – this is an electrical stimulus applied, which is at least 20 to 25% above that necessary for a maximal response.

Ideal nerve stimulator
1. The stimulus should produce a monophasic, rectangular wave (a square wave). Biphasic pulses may cause a burst of action potentials in a nerve – repetitive firing – and so increase the response of the nerve to the stimulation.
2. The duration of the pulse should not exceed 0.2–0.3 ms.
3. A constant current stimulation is preferred to a constant voltage stimulation as current determines the stimulation of the nerve.
4. It should be battery operated and generate no more that 80 mA.
5. It should have a built in warming device. During cooling, skin resistance increases up to 5000 ohms and causes a decrease in current delivered to a nerve, which may fall below the supramaximal level.

6. The polarity of the electrodes should be indicated.
7. The apparatus should be capable of delivering the following modes of stimulus.
   - TOF, single, and repetitive mode
   - Single twitch stimulus at 0.1–1.0 Hz
   - Tetanic stimulus at 50 Hz
   - Built in time constant systems to facilitate post tetanic count
   - Double burst capacity

A 76. **A.** false **B.** false **C.** false **D.** false **E.** true

The depth of the burnt area may be increased by infection. There is a risk of infection spreading to become systemic sepsis with ARDS and multi-organ failure.

Patients at risk from sepsis are those who have lost their protective skin barrier and those who are immune suppressed.

Measures to reduce the risk of infection include:
- Nurse in a clean area
- Take measures to avoid cross infection
- Use topical antimicrobial prophylaxis
- Antibiotic cover is necessary to cover dressing changes

A 77. **A.** false **B.** true **C.** true **D.** true **E.** false

Clonidine is an imidazole with α-2 adrenergic agonist activity. It was originally introduced as an antihypertensive. Its main clinical role is now related to use as an adjuvant to analgesics and anaesthetics – to decrease anaesthetic requirements and to attenuate sympathetic excitatory responses in patients undergoing general anaesthesia.

The action of clonidine on α-2 receptors, which are widely distributed throughout the CNS and the body results in:
- Sedation and anxiolysis
- Antisialogogue effects
- Analgesia – supraspinal and spinal
- It enhances conduction blockade by local anaesthetics
- It reduces the requirement for general anaesthetic agents
- It decreases intraocular pressure
- It stops shivering postoperatively

Peripheral and central effects on the CVS

- Inhibition of noradrenaline release from prejunctional nerve endings
- Hypotensive and bradycardiac effects produced centrally
- Anti-arrhythmic effects mediated by the vagus nerve

Diffuse action on hormone function

- Reduces thyroid function
- Reduces sympathetic outflow
- Reduces the stress induced ACTH and cortisol release
- Increased secretion of growth hormone

A **78.** **A.** true **B.** false **C.** true **D.** true **E.** true

Normal blood lactate is 0.6 to 1.2 mmol/l and levels above 5 mmol/l cause a significant acidosis. Concentrations greater than 9 mmol/l carry an 80% mortality rate.

Lactate is made in skeletal muscle and red blood cells. When oxygen supplies are limited pyruvate is reduced to NADH to form lactate. The reaction is catalysed by lactate dehydrogenase.

The importance of this reaction is that it produces two molecules of ATP.

It regenerates NAD^+, which sustains continued glycolysis in skeletal muscle and erythrocytes under anaerobic conditions.

The limiting factor is the liver, which must oxidise lactate back to pyruvate for subsequent gluconeogenesis in the Cori cycle. This pathway merely buys time during periods of anaerobic metabolism.

A **79.** **A.** false **B.** false **C.** true **D.** true **E.** true

Until recently a low dose dopamine infusion (1 to 3 μg/kg/min) was the most popular treatment for oliguria in the presence of an adequate circulating volume. The increase in renal blood flow was thought to be due to a specific effect mediated through dopamine receptors. In reality this dose of dopamine has a significant inotropic and chronotropic effect and the increase in blood flow is probably secondary to a general increase in cardiac output. Dopamine may also induce gut mucosal ischaemia. Like frusemide, dopamine will often induce a diuresis but has not been shown to be protective against acute renal failure.

Paper 2

Answers

A 80. **A.** true **B.** false **C.** true **D.** false **E.** true

The appropriate values are:

Umbilical vein

- PO_2 – 4 kPa
- PCO_2 – 6 kPa
- pH – 7.2

Umbilical artery

- PO_2 – 2 kPa
- PCO_2 – 7 kPa

The uterine artery CO_2 will be less than 5 kPa because of maternal hyperventilation.

A 81. **A.** true **B.** true **C.** false **D.** false **E.** true

The algorithm for the management of broad complex tachycardia includes:

No pulse – use VF protocol.

Pulse present but BP <90 mmHg, chest pain, heart failure rate >150 bpm – synchronised DC shock 100, 200, 360 J or equivalent biphasic energy. Correct low potassium, amiodarone 150 mg iv over 10 min.

Pulse not present – correct low potassium, amiodarone 150 mg iv over 10 min, or lidocaine 50 mg iv over 2 min and repeat up to 200 mg in 5 min. Then synchronised DC shock. Further amiodarone 150 mg iv over 10 min then 300 mg over 1 h.

A 82. **A.** true **B.** true **C.** false **D.** false **E.** false

A coeliac plexus block can be used to treat the pain of chronic pancreatitis. Thoracic epidurals are also effective if there is no contraindication.

A 83. **A.** true **B.** true **C.** true **D.** true **E.** false

Phantom limb pain is a chronic pain perceived in an absent body part. The incidence varies greatly from 15–100%. It can occur in all ages with a peak of 100% at age 8. Phantom limb pain can be associated with stump pain, which is a chronic pain perceived in the amputation stump. The incidence of stump pain is 10 to 25%.

It may be diffuse and is often associated with a palpable stump neuroma. This makes fitting a limb prosthesis difficult.

It is uncertain whether the source of the phantom sensation is a central or spinal phenomenon. It is most likely central due to the intact body normogram on the cerebral cortex. Lesions or interventions affecting the spinal cord or brain can abolish phantom sensations but do not necessarily eliminate the phantom limb pain.

Treatment
Elimination of the pain and sensation can be extremely difficult. Measures include:
- Anticonvulsant therapies – carbamazepine, gabapentine
- Tricyclic-antidepressants – amitriptyline
- TENS
- Spinal cord stimulation
- The wearing of the prosthesis and increased mobility despite initial pain

Probably the most progressive treatment is the use of pre-emptive analgesia before amputation. The theory is to desensitise the proposed body part for at least 48 h before amputation. This is an option for the atraumatic amputation. For lower limbs, an epidural infusion has been used for upper limbs and brachial plexus block or stellate ganglion block has been used with good effect.

A 84. **A.** true **B.** true **C.** false **D.** true **E.** false

The most important factors affecting the spread of spinal anaesthetic are:
- The tonicity of the solution
- The position of the patient

Less important factors include:
- The site of the injection
- Speed of injection and barbotage
- Dose of drug
- Volume of anaesthetic
- Age of patient
- Height of patient
- Weight of patient
- Smaller space such as in pregnancy

The duration of the block depends on:

- The dose of the drug
- Tonicity of the anaesthetic solution
- The protein binding of the drug – bupivacaine acts longer than lidocaine

A 85. A. false **B.** false **C.** true **D.** false **E.** true

The following factors speed up the rate of induction with inhalational agents:

1. Increased inspired concentrations. The higher the concentration the higher the level achieved in blood.
2. Increased alveolar ventilation. Increasing alveolar minute volume speeds up the approximation of alveolar to inspired levels.
3. Small FRC.
4. Low blood to gas partition coefficient. A low blood to gas partition coefficient indicates low solubility in blood so equilibrium will be rapid.
5. Second gas effect.
   Administration of a rapidly absorbed gas given in high concentration (typically N_2O) together with a volatile agent of lower solubility – produces an increasing alveolar concentration of the second agent thus promoting its absorption.
6. Low cardiac output.
   This will cause more rapid increase in the pulmonary arterial concentration of a volatile agent and permit inspired and arterial tensions to equalise sooner. So the rate of induction is increased.

A 86. A. false **B.** true **C.** false **D.** true **E.** true

Enteral nutrition can be given by:

- Nasogastric tube
- Naso-jejunal tube
- Percutaneous gastrostomy tube
- Percutaneous jejunostomy tube

Post pyloric feeding is becoming more popular as gastric atony can be a problem in the critically ill patient. Give 30–40 kcal/kg/day with vitamins and minerals. Need more than 25 cm of ileum, which is intact and functioning.

Advantages of enteral route

- Cheaper, no risk of disconnection, physiological, protects gut from erosions by physical barrier and increases splanchnic blood flow
- Reduces villous atrophy, reduces nosocomial pneumonia, reduces translocation of toxins across the gut wall
- Reduces incidence of a calculus cholecystitis
- Enhances secretion of IgA
- Supports the normal gut flora. Reduces bacterial translocation and reduces risk of gram negative sepsis
- Fewer metabolic complications
- No associated complications such as tube sepsis, blockage, and displacement

Contraindications

- Intestinal obstruction
- High gut fistula
- Recent upper gastrointestinal anastomosis
- Pancreatitis is an indication for nasojejunal (post pyloric) feeding

A **87.** **A.** false **B.** false **C.** true **D.** false **E.** false

The recommendations intended to promote maximum electrical safety are:

- Use battery powered equipment wherever possible
- Earth all enclosures
- Isolate all circuits attached to the patient
- Use a high impedance input between the patient and the device – i.e. the use of isolating capacitors in diathermy equipment is due to the fact that capacitors have a high impedance to a low frequency (50 Hz) current, but a low impedance to a high (1 MHz) frequency current
- Arrange regular maintenance and testing by qualified staff

A **88.** **A.** false **B.** false **C.** false **D.** true **E.** false

The physiological impact of a spinal block is proportional to its dermatological height. Blockade of the sympathetic nerves arising from the mid-thoracic and upper thoracic segments causes significant venous pooling and results in hypotension.

- A spinal block to T10 has a minimum cardiovascular impact
- A spinal block to T6 causes a decrease in arterial blood pressure in the region of 25%

- A block to T4 decreases blood pressure by 30%
- The cardiac sympathetic nerve have roots values of T1 to T4. Blockade of these nerves causes bradycardia and hypotension
- Unopposed parasympathetic activity in the gut can cause hyper-peristalsis with blocks above T5, which are often associated with nausea and vomiting
- Extension of the block to the mid cervical region C3 to C5 affects the roots of the phrenic nerve
- Extension of the local anaesthetic through the foramen magnum allows it around the hind brain and causes loss of consciousness – often called a total spinal

A **89.** **A.** true **B.** false **C.** false **D.** false **E.** false

Most dental procedures can be performed under local anaesthesia and it is recommended that general anaesthesia is limited to the following groups:

1. Patients who are unable to co-operate because of immaturity or physical or mental disability.
2. Patients in whom local anaesthesia has proven unsuccessful or is unlikely to be completely effective due to the extent of the surgery or the presence of infection or the number of quadrants to be operated on.
3. Patients with a history suggestive of hypersensitivity or allergy to the contents of the local anaesthetic ampoule.
4. Patients who suffer from extreme nervousness and who prefer to undergo any form of dental treatment while unaware.

Ambulatory dental anaesthesia is usually limited to patients assessed as ASA 1 to 3 but can include other patients when undertaken in a district hospital.

A **90.** **A.** true **B.** false **C.** false **D.** false **E.** false

Answers

Question	A	B	C	D	E
1	T	T	T	F	F
2	F	F	F	T	F
3	T	F	F	F	F
4	T	F	F	F	T
5	T	F	T	T	T
6	F	T	F	T	T
7	F	T	F	F	T
8	T	T	F	F	F
9	F	F	T	T	T
10	T	T	T	F	F
11	T	F	T	T	F
12	F	T	T	F	T
13	T	T	T	F	T
14	F	T	F	F	T
15	T	T	T	F	F
16	F	F	T	F	F
17	F	F	F	F	F
18	T	T	F	T	F
19	T	F	T	F	F
20	T	F	T	T	T
21	T	T	T	T	T
22	T	T	T	F	T
23	T	F	F	F	F
24	T	T	F	F	F
25	F	F	F	T	F
26	F	T	T	T	T
27	T	F	T	T	F
28	T	T	T	F	F
29	T	T	T	T	F
30	F	T	F	T	T

Question	A	B	C	D	E
31	T	F	T	F	T
32	T	F	T	T	T
33	T	F	T	T	T
34	F	F	T	F	T
35	T	T	F	T	F
36	F	F	T	T	T
37	T	T	F	T	T
38	F	F	T	T	T
39	T	T	T	T	T
40	T	T	T	F	F
41	T	F	F	F	T
42	T	T	F	F	T
43	F	F	T	T	T
44	F	F	T	F	F
45	T	F	F	T	T
46	T	F	F	T	T
47	T	F	T	T	F
48	T	F	T	T	T
49	F	T	F	T	T
50	T	T	T	T	T
51	T	F	F	T	T
52	F	F	F	T	T
53	F	F	T	F	T
54	F	T	F	F	T
55	T	T	F	T	F
56	T	T	T	F	T
57	T	T	T	T	F
58	T	F	F	F	F
59	T	T	F	F	F
60	T	F	T	F	F

Question	A	B	C	D	E
61	F	F	F	T	T
62	T	F	T	F	F
63	T	T	T	F	T
64	T	F	T	T	F
65	F	F	T	F	T
66	F	T	F	T	T
67	T	T	F	F	T
68	T	F	T	T	T
69	T	F	T	T	F
70	F	F	F	F	T
71	T	T	F	F	F
72	F	T	T	T	T
73	T	T	F	F	F
74	F	F	T	F	T
75	F	F	F	F	F
76	F	F	F	F	T
77	F	T	T	T	F
78	T	F	T	T	T
79	F	F	T	T	T
80	T	F	T	F	T
81	T	T	F	F	T
82	T	T	F	F	F
83	T	T	T	T	F
84	T	T	F	T	F
85	F	F	T	F	T
86	F	T	F	T	T
87	F	F	T	F	F
88	F	F	F	T	F
89	T	F	F	F	F
90	T	F	F	F	F

Paper 3 Answers

A 1. **A.** true **B.** false **C.** false **D.** false **E.** true

In pregnancy the FRC is reduced by pressure on the diaphragm. But the total lung capacity is increased. Airway resistance reduces as smooth muscle relaxes. The maternal arterial carbon dioxide tension is reduced while the oxygen tension increases.

A 2. **A.** true **B.** true **C.** true **D.** true **E.** false

Chronic renal failure and uraemia may lead to fluid overload and a large heart, cardiac tamponade, hypertension and uraemic pericarditis.

A 3. **A.** true **B.** true **C.** true **D.** true **E.** false

Transoesophageal echocardiography can be likened to an internal stethoscope. It will look at myocardial wall contractility, valve function and blood flow through the valves and septal wall activity. It can be used to gauge blood flow but cannot measure flow precisely or measure pressures.

A 4. **A.** false **B.** false **C.** false **D.** false **E.** true

This patient has a low oxygen tension and a low carbon dioxide. The pH is normal so there is a compensation for a long-standing condition in which oxygenation is reduced. There is neither alkalosis, nor hypoventilation as the carbon dioxide is low.

A 5. **A.** false **B.** true **C.** true **D.** false **E.** true

The postoperative phase is characterised by a negative nitrogen balance in which nitrogen is anabolised at the rate of 3–5 g/day.

Protein has a calorific value of 4 cal/g (the same as carbohydrate). 1 g of nitrogen equates with 6.25 g of protein.

Grams of protein required = urinary nitrogen × 6.25. Most protein contains 16% nitrogen. Urinary urea makes up 80–90% of the total urinary nitrogen. Potassium excretion is a minimum, obligatory 1 mmol/kg.

A 6. **A.** true **B.** false **C.** false **D.** false **E.** false

The lipid solubility of volatile agents is directly related to potency. The mechanism of action proposed by the Overton Meyer theory is no longer valid. The action of volatile agents is more complicated than simple fat solubility, involving the lipid and protein components of the cell membranes.

A 7. **A.** true **B.** false **C.** true **D.** false **E.** true

Pulmonary oedema takes time to develop and is not immediate. Smoke injury is not associated with heat injury as the smoke will have cooled by the time it reaches the lung.

A 8. **A.** true **B.** true **C.** false **D.** false **E.** true

Chronic obstructive airways disease is chronic airways obstruction, or asthma which leads to emphysema. Type 1 respiratory failure is hyperventilation creating a low carbon dioxide tension while trying to maintain a normal oxygen tension. Type 2 respiratory failure is described when the carbon dioxide tension rises and the oxygen tension falls. The patient is dependent on a hypoxic drive for respiration combined with the raised carbon dioxide tension. In Type 2 failure giving bicarbonate will increase the carbon dioxide tension and kill the patient. The bicarbonate rises to compensate for the rise in carbon dioxide to return the pH to near normal. Bear in mind that venous oxygen tension is normally 5.3 kPa and is 75% saturated with oxygen.

A 9. **A.** true **B.** false **C.** true **D.** true **E.** true

A narrow cuff acts as a tourniquet and over reads. Doppler shift is the change in frequency of the returning sound wave due to the flow of the fluid.

Paper 3 Answers

A 10. **A.** false **B.** false **C.** true **D.** true **E.** true

Sickle cell trait is the heterozygous state. The amount of HbS is usually about 40%. So sickling is uncommon but can occur. It does not lead to a severe anaemia.

Electrophoresis of plasma proteins detects HbS and is the means of diagnosis. Sickle trait does not normally lead to sickling but sickling can occur in very extreme anoxic conditions such as problems with anaesthesia or altitude. Then haemolysis will occur – but this is very rare. (This is a difficult answer to be certain of the meaning.)

Haemolysis can occur in sickle disease on exposure to drugs, acute infections and associated G6PD deficiency.

A 11. **A.** false **B.** false **C.** true **D.** true **E.** true

It is a narrowing of the aorta. Two forms exist. Infantile is preductal. The commoner adult type occurs at or distal to the ductus arteriosus. 80% are associated with a bicuspid aortic valve. It is associated with Turner's syndrome.

X-ray finding show typical notching of the lower margins of the 5th, 6th and 7th ribs due to increased blood flow through intercostal arteries. There may be post-stenotic dilatation of the aorta.

There is hypertension in the upper body and limbs leading to headache and nosebleeds. There is poor blood flow in the lower limbs with coldness and claudication in the legs.

A 12. **A.** true **B.** false **C.** true **D.** false **E.** false

Hypokalaemia leads to flattening or inversion of the T waves, prominent U waves, ST segment depression and a prolonged PR interval. There is muscle weakness and reduced cardiac contractility.

Hyperkalaemia leads to high T waves, wide QRS complex, prolonged PR interval and loss of P waves, loss of R height and ST depression.

Wolf-Parkinson-White syndrome gives δ waves.

A 13. **A.** false **B.** false **C.** false **D.** true **E.** false

Acute tubular necrosis is due to reduced oxygenation of the kidney. Glomerular surface area is reduced and so filtration is reduced. There is patchy tubular necrosis with reduced reabsorption, but these cells recover rapidly. The tubular lumen is also affected by obstruction caused by the debris shed from damaged tubular cells.

The features of renal failure include a raised creatinine and raised potassium.

Initially the volume of urine will be low with an osmolarity equal to plasma (not concentrated) as a glomerular filtrate is passed.

A 14. **A.** true **B.** true **C.** false **D.** false **E.** true

Single blind is the subject unaware of the treatment, double blind is the investigator and subject unaware of the treatment.

Observe bias can still come into double blind studies.

A 15. **A.** true **B.** true **C.** false **D.** true **E.** false

There is a large baby but not due to the effects of maternal insulin.

A 16. **A.** false **B.** false **C.** true **D.** false **E.** false

Clomipramine is a tricyclic antidepressant, like amitriptyline, which inhibits the re-uptake of catecholamines as well as serotonin.

The mechanisms of action of sympathomimetics are divided into α 1 and 2 and β 1 and 2.

Stimulation of β-receptors through coupling to the enzyme adenyl cyclase, leads to the production of cyclic monophosphate (cAMP).

α-receptor activity alters membrane transfer of calcium, which leads to actions such as smooth muscle contraction.

Drugs act by:

- Direct action on receptors – adrenaline, isoprenaline
- Indirectly by releasing adrenaline – amphetamine, ephedrine
- Both direct and indirect – dopamine

A 17. **A.** true **B.** true **C.** true **D.** true **E.** false

Drugs cross the placenta under a concentration gradient. The amount of free drug in the plasma available to pass depends on protein binding. More of a drug will pass if it has a low molecular size and no electrical charge.

A 18. **A.** true **B.** false **C.** false **D.** false **E.** false

The Fick principle for measuring cardiac output depends on injecting a solution of known temperature and measuring the change in temperature at the catheter tip. The patient's temperature is not relevant.

The proximal lumen should be at a place where mixed venous blood is present. There should be a whole heart chamber between the proximal port and the distal probe.

A 19. **A.** false **B.** false **C.** true **D.** true **E.** false

Occurs from the medial wall and Little's area. Epistaxis may indicate hypertension and if bleeding is severe may result in anaemia. Ligation of a branch of the carotid artery may be relevant to stop bleeding. The facial artery and the sphenopalatine arteries supply the septum.

A 20. **A.** true **B.** true **C.** false **D.** true **E.** true

This is a condition of neurofibromas and pigmentation. The neurofibromas arise from the neurilemma sheath. On the skin there are café-au-lait brown marks. The neurofibromas act as space occupying lesions, which may cause paraplegia and deafness.

Associated conditions include:

- Pulmonary fibrosis
- Cardiomyopathy
- Scoliosis
- Renal artery stenosis
- Phaeochromocytoma
- Fibrous dysplasia of bone

A 21. **A.** false **B.** true **C.** false **D.** true **E.** false

Blood flow in the microcirculation is less homogeneous. Pulmonary artery catheters do not assess the microcirculation.

White cells will alter viscosity. The permeability of the membrane will not alter blood flow.

A **22.** **A.** true **B.** true **C.** false **D.** true **E.** false

The oxygen concentrator removes nitrogen from air. They can be used anywhere where there is supply of electricity. The argon will be concentrated in the resulting gas and so will be higher than the 0.8% in air. The nitrogen can be driven out of the zeolite by heating and so it can be regenerated.

A **23.** **A.** true **B.** false **C.** false **D.** true **E.** false

Oxygen and nitric oxide are paramagnetic gases.

A **24.** **A.** true **B.** false **C.** true **D.** false **E.** true

Porphyrias are a group of inherited diseases in which there is an abnormality of haem synthesis. This results in an excess production of porphyrins. These are made of four pyrrole rings.

Alcohol, barbiturates, oral contraceptives and a large number of lipid soluble drugs can precipitate acute intermittent porphyria. A safe anaesthetic can be given with opioids such as morphine and fentanyl, benzodiazepines, muscle relaxants and volatile agents.

Dehydration must be avoided.

A **25.** **A.** false **B.** false **C.** false **D.** false **E.** false

The valve is normally 5 cm^2. At 1 cm^2 the stenosis is severe. Left atrial pressure rises, which gives rise to a large left atrium. Symptoms appear at 2 cm^2. The pulse is small volume and atrial fibrillation may develop. When pulmonary hypertension develops the "a" wave of the jugular pulse will be prominent. The apex beat is tapping due to a palpable first heart sound and rotation backward of the left ventricle. The larger right ventricle gives a para sternal heave. On auscultation the first heart sound is loud until there is calcification in the mitral valve, when there is no noise. The opening snap is due to sudden opening of the mitral valve due to the force of the atrial pressure.

The closeness of the opening snap to the second heart sound is proportional to the severity of the stenosis. The length of the mid diastolic murmur is proportional to the severity of the stenosis. The severity of disease is also related to the development of pulmonary hypertension. This leads to pulmonary regurgitation and an early diastolic pulmonary murmur (Graham-Steele murmur).

A 26. **A.** false **B.** false **C.** false **D.** true **E.** false

Sevoflurane boils at 49°C, SVP at 20°C 33 kPa.

Sevoflurane has a blood gas partition coefficient of 0.6 and reacts with soda lime to produce Compound A.

A 27. **A.** false **B.** false **C.** false **D.** true **E.** true

Hospital acquired infection is best prevented by hand washing and a good space between beds.

Isolation of patients should reduce the spread of infectious diseases. Separation of patients would be expected to reduce the spread of hospital-acquired infections.

A 28. **A.** false **B.** true **C.** true **D.** false **E.** true

Trigeminal neuralgia is not associated with any abnormal function of the trigeminal nerve. It is approached through the foramen ovale, which is the exit for the mandibular branch through the floor of the cranium.

A 29. **A.** false **B.** true **C.** true **D.** false **E.** true

Malignant hyperpyrexia is an autosomal dominant condition. The incidence is about 1 in 15,000 in children, 1 in 25,000 in adults. It is associated with a defect in calcium release from the sarcoplasmic reticulum.

It is more common in males but not due to a sex linked gene. It can be precipitated by suxamethonium or a volatile agent. Stress precipitates a similar condition in pigs.

The condition is linked to various muscular dystrophies including Duchenne dystrophy.

A 30. **A.** true **B.** true **C.** false **D.** false **E.** true

TURP syndrome is associated with absorption of water from the bladder. This leads to water intoxication and dilution of the plasma electrolytes.

The condition is easier to detect, but not prevented by regional anaesthesia. Treatment involves hypertonic saline and removal of water by a diuretic.

A 31. **A.** true **B.** true **C.** false **D.** false **E.** false

Penicillins are bactericidal, acting on cell wall synthesis. They are most effective on cells that are dividing.

A 32. **A.** true **B.** true **C.** false **D.** false **E.** true

Cerebral blood flow (CBF) is 50 ml/100 g. Autoregulation means that as the blood flow increases the blood vessels will constrict and vice versa. This occurs within the range of mean arterial pressures of 60 and 130 mmHg. So 50–100 is within this range. Autoregulation is shifted to the right in hypertensive patients (90–160 mmHg). Autoregulation is reduced or abolished in hypoxia, hypercapnia, acute brain disease and trauma. Breathing 100% oxygen reduces it.

CBF increases with rising carbon dioxide tension. The greatest change occurs around a normal $pPaCO_2$ when a change of 1 kPa will alter CBF by 30%.

Mannitol will increase cardiac output, which will alter CBF.

A 33. **A.** true **B.** false **C.** false **D.** true **E.** true

Posteriorly the nerves lie between the pleura and the posterior intercostal membrane. The nerves pass between the intercostalis internus muscle and the innermost muscle layer which is subcostalis posteriorly and intercostalis intimus laterally. Under the rib the relationship from below upwards is nerve, artery and then vein.

The branches of each nerve are the collateral, lateral and the anterior nerve of the thorax as well as a branch that innervates the intercostal muscles.

A 34. **A.** false **B.** false **C.** true **D.** false **E.** true

The right ventricular pressure is high (normal 40/8). Pulmonary artery pressure is high (normal 25/10). The wedge pressure is normal. He has pulmonary hypertension, possibly due to a VSD with a left to right shunt.

A 35. **A.** true **B.** true **C.** true **D.** false **E.** false

Sodium is low, potassium is high. This can occur in oliguric renal failure with water retention, or with a lack of adrenocorticotrophic hormone or glucocorticoids as found in pituitary or adrenal insufficiency.

A 36. **A.** true **B.** false **C.** true **D.** false **E.** false

The risk of central venous catheter infection is less when the internal jugular is used and with materials that are less likely to form thrombus or are impregnated to counteract infection. The amount of handling and the number of times the site is injected into or otherwise disturbed increases the risk of infection.

A 37. **A.** true **B.** true **C.** true **D.** false **E.** false

Haemophilus influenzae type B causes epiglottitis. The condition is unusual over the age of 5 years. The onset is sudden with high fever. Prevention is now by vaccination. Treatment is with intravenous ceftazidine or chloramphenicol.

Acute laryngotracheobronchitis is a complication of an upper respiratory tract infection.

The vocal cords in epiglottitis are oedematous leading to narrowing laryngeal stridor, hoarse voice and a barking cough (or croup). Treatment is humidification and oxygen. Intubation may be necessary.

A 38. **A.** true **B.** true **C.** true **D.** true **E.** true

The Portal vein is about 8 cm long. Obstruction may produce ascites, whether the obstruction is intra- or extra-hepatic.

A 39. **A.** false **B.** false **C.** false **D.** false **E.** false

Initially 100% oxygen would be best with a low respiratory rate and a long expiratory phase. The patient will be generating his or her own PEEP so it is better to minimise any expiratory resistance.

The peak inspiratory flow rate should be set to maximise the tidal volume.

A 40. **A.** true **B.** true **C.** false **D.** false **E.** true

Physiological oliguria is usually defined as <300 ml of urine in 24 h. It occurs with normal renal function in hypotension and hypovolaemia and a need to conserve water. The urine is concentrated with an osmolarity greater than plasma (plasma osmolarity 300 mosmol/l) + 100 mosmol/l, or a specific gravity >1.020. The U:P osmolarity ratio is high 2:1.

- The urine sodium is low (<20 mmol/l)
- The U:P urea ratio is high (20)
- The U:P creatinine ratio is high (40)

In intrinsic renal failure the specific gravity is fixed at 1.01–1.02.

- Urine sodium is high (>40 mmol/l)
- U:P urea is low (10)
- U:P creatinine is low (10)
- The U:P osmolarity is low (<serum + 100 mosmol/l)

A 41. **A.** true **B.** true **C.** true **D.** false **E.** true

The pulmonary artery may enlarge in response to an increased blood flow. Fallot's tetralogy is an overriding aorta with pulmonary stenosis.

A 42. **A.** true **B.** true **C.** true **D.** false **E.** false

Hypothermia is frequently lethal when the core temperature falls below 32°C. Consciousness is impaired at 30°C. Conduction through the heart is slowed. Ventricular arrhythmias occur at 30°C and ventricular fibrillation occurs at 28°C. J waves – rounded waves above the isoelectric line – appear after the QRS.

A 43. **A.** false **B.** true **C.** false **D.** true **E.** false

The tests for brainstem death should be made by two people with experience in the field, one of whom should be a consultant.

The cause of the coma must be known. The patient must be apnoeic and must not be affected by a reversible cause of brain stem depression such as drugs, alcohol, hypothermia or metabolic and endocrine disturbances.

The apnoea test is performed after pre-oxygenation with 100% oxygen for some 5 min. The patient is observed for 10 min after the ventilator has been turned off. The carbon dioxide during and after the 10 min should be at a level to induce respiration of 6.7 kPa (50 mmHg).

A **44.** **A.** false **B.** false **C.** false **D.** false **E.** false

Tramadol is an agonist at μ, δ and κ receptors. It inhibits noradrenaline uptake but enhances 5-HT release.

A **45.** **A.** false **B.** true **C.** false **D.** false **E.** false

The molecular size of albumin is 35,000 daltons. It is made in the liver with the other proteins (except γ globulins, which are produced in the reticuloendothelial system). 10–12 g are made daily.

A **46.** **A.** true **B.** false **C.** true **D.** true **E.** true

Patients with blood group A carry antigen A, which is found in saliva and gastric juice in about 80% who have a secretor gene.

The most common blood groups are O (44%) and A (45%) with B (8%) and AB (3%).

A **47.** **A.** true **B.** true **C.** true **D.** true **E.** true

A **48.** **A.** true **B.** false **C.** false **D.** false **E.** false

The type B non-fighter (blue bloater) respiratory failure do not appear breathless but have

- Marked arterial hypoxaemia $PaO_2 < 8$ kPa
- Marked CO_2 retention $PaCO_2 > 8$ kPa
- Secondary polycythaemia
- Cor pulmonale

A **49.** **A.** false **B.** false **C.** true **D.** false **E.** true

High frequency ventilation is one of a number of options. Steroids are not of proven benefit. Albumin is not essential and may lead to alveolar proteinosis if albumin leaks into the lung.

A 50. **A.** true **B.** false **C.** false **D.** false **E.** true

PEFR varies with the time of day, as do other physiological parameters. The Vitalograph is used to measure FVC and FEV1. To measure PEFR, a Wright's peak flow meter is needed or a pneumotacograph.

A 51. **A.** false **B.** false **C.** true **D.** false **E.** false

Acromegaly is due to a pituitary tumour. Growth hormone is usually low. IGF-1 is raised. The glucose tolerance test shows diabetes mellitus in 25% of cases. The pituitary adenoma displaces normal pituitary tissue leading to hypopituitarism. About a third of cases have hyperprolactinaemia.

Without treatment death occurs early due to heart failure, coronary artery disease and the effects of hypertension. Conn's syndrome is due to adrenal hyperplasia or an adrenal adenoma.

A 52. **A.** false **B.** false **C.** false **D.** true **E.** true

Carcinoid tumours originate from the enterochromaffin cells of the intestine. They secrete serotonin (5-HT), bradykinin, histamine and tachykinins – also substance P, prostaglandins and histamine. The serotonin causes diarrhoea and the kinins lead to flushing.

A 53. **A.** false **B.** false **C.** true **D.** false **E.** false

Endotoxin is a lipopolysaccharide derived from the cell wall of gram-negative bacteria, which is an important trigger for septic shock. The Limulus crab is used as a test for endotoxin.

A 54. **A.** false **B.** true **C.** false **D.** true **E.** true

A rise in serum amylase occurs in a number of abdominal emergencies such as cholecystitis and perforated peptic ulcer. A level of five times or more above the normal is very likely to be pancreatitis.

Indications of severity and a poor outcome in the first 48 h are:

- Age >50
- WBC $>15 \times 10^9$/l
- Blood glucose >10 mmol/l

Paper 3 Answers

- Serum urea >16 mmol/l
- Serum albumin <30 g/l
- Serum aminotransferase >200 IU/l
- Serum calcium <2 mmol/l
- Serum LDH >600 IU/l
- PaO_2 <8.0 kPa
- Base deficit of >4 meq/l
- BUN >5 mg/100 ml
- Estimated fluid sequestration >6 l

A 55. **A.** false **B.** true **C.** true **D.** false **E.** true

Patient controlled analgesia is not patient controlled if there is a continuous infusion.

Respiratory depression will occur with larger doses of morphine, with added sedative drugs and when an epidural or other local anaesthetic block becomes effective in relieving the pain in the presence of systemic opioids.

A 56. **A.** true **B.** true **C.** true **D.** false **E.** true

In crush syndrome, a high urine output is desirable to maintain tubular flow.

A 57. **A.** true **B.** true **C.** true **D.** true **E.** false

Wind up is a term used to describe an abnormal process in which the normal painful sensation gets worse in the absence of any additional injury.

It is associated with an augmented action in the substantia gelatinosa and is inhibited by NMDA antagonists. While morphine has some effect opioids like methadone and tramadol are more effective NMDA antagonists.

A 58. **A.** true **B.** true **C.** true **D.** false **E.** false

Ergometrine is reversed by:

- Myometrial muscle relaxants
- Salbutamol – a β-2 agonist, ritodrine a β-2 agonist used to inhibit premature labour (also terbutaline)
- Isoflurane has a direct action on uterine muscle

A 59. **A.** true **B.** false **C.** false **D.** false **E.** true

The use of routine investigation without an indication is not recommended, as it is not cost effective.

A CXR is not useful in patients without symptoms. CXR should be considered in high-risk patients – those with possible metastases of carcinoma indicated by symptoms, signs or weight loss and those from high-risk areas of diseases such as tuberculosis, preferably with symptoms.

A 60. **A.** true **B.** true **C.** false **D.** true **E.** true

Blood can be returned into cold store within 30 min of being taken into a room temperature.

A 61. **A.** false **B.** false **C.** true **D.** false **E.** false

EMLA is 2.5% lidocaine and 2.5% prilocaine.

This mixture of two local anaesthetics changes the melting point of the local anaesthetics. This phenomenon is called a eutectic mixture.

A 62. **A.** true **B.** true **C.** false **D.** false **E.** false

The complications of chronic renal failure include:
- Anaemia
- Renal osteodystrophy, including hyperparathyroidism
- Pruritus
- Reduced gastric emptying
- Gout
- Reduced insulin elimination by the kidney
- Autonomic dysfunction

The excretion of many drugs such as digoxin is delayed.

A 63. **A.** false **B.** false **C.** true **D.** false **E.** true

Addison's disease is a reduction in adrenal cortical function.

The features include:
- Hypovolaemia due to deficiency of mineralocorticoid and hypotension and pigmentation

- Blood may show low sodium, high potassium and low glucose
- Salt and water balances are impaired due to lack of fludrocortisone and mineralocorticoid

ACTH has no benefit as there is reduced adrenal function.

A **64.** **A.** false **B.** true **C.** true **D.** false **E.** true

Hepatitis C is an RNA virus, responsible for most cases of hepatitis infection following blood transfusion. Over 50% of cases go on to develop chronic liver disease. Cirrhosis develops in 20–30%, of which 15% develop hepatocellular carcinoma.

A **65.** **A.** true **B.** true **C.** true **D.** true **E.** true

Haemoptysis is a sign of:

- Mitral stenosis due to the raised venous pressure from the high left atrial pressure
- Good Pasteur syndrome is a type II cytotoxic hypersensitivity reaction mediated by anti-GBM antibody – presents with severe haemoptysis and glomerulonephritis
- Wegener's granulomatosis – a vasculitis of unknown origin. Lesions affect the lungs, and kidneys. There is cough, haemoptysis and pleuritic pain
- Behcet's disease is a systemic vasculitis of unknown origin presenting with oral ulceration
- Bronchiectasis is dilatation of the larger airways usually following a severe pneumonia. These damaged airways are very susceptible to repeated infection

A **66.** **A.** true **B.** true **C.** false **D.** true **E.** true

Jaundiced patients are susceptible to hepatic-renal failure. Either mannitol or a diuretic should be given to ensure a good urine flow.

Clotting may be affected by vitamin K deficiency. All patients having major surgery should have anti-thrombosis prophylaxis.

A **67.** **A.** false **B.** true **C.** true **D.** true **E.** true

Bronchogenic carcinomas may present with lung symptoms, metastatic disease to tissues such as bone or non-metastatic conditions.

The non-metastatic presentations include:

- Hypertrophic pulmonary osteoarthropathy with joint stiffness
- ACTH syndrome
- Inappropriate ADH syndrome
- Hypercalcaemia
- Hypoglycaemia
- Thyrotoxicosis

Horner's syndrome will be produced by pressure from an apical tumour.

A 68. A. false **B.** true **C.** false **D.** false **E.** true

The initial phase, which lasts minutes, is of intense neural activity and raised BP. The next phase of spinal shock is marked by lack of autonomic control. This can last up to 8 weeks. There is low BP, cooling due to vasodilation, loss of muscle tone and reflexes and excess of vagal tone may lead to bradycardia or cardiac arrest.

Other changes include:

- The muscles undergo changes following denervation – the motor end plate extends to cover the muscle cell membrane. Suxamethonium causes widespread depolarisation and the release of more potassium than normal
- Urinary retention requiring catheterisation

After some weeks, reflex movement of the legs is possible with recovery of spinal reflexes leading to increased muscle tone, reflexes and muscle spasm. Extensor spasm in the legs is dominant, the extensors being stronger than the leg flexor muscles. Sympathetic activity also returns.

A 69. A. false **B.** false **C.** true **D.** true **E.** false

Myotonia means that muscle contraction persists. In dystrophia myotonica, the contraction continues after giving neuromuscular blocking drugs, local anaesthetics and following nerve section.

The distal and cranial muscles are most affected. The grip does not relax. Cardiac conduction is impaired leading to sudden death. The myotonia may be improved by warmth and class I anti-arrhythmics such as phenytoin and procainamide. Respiratory muscle involvement leads to hypoventilation.

A 70. **A.** true **B.** true **C.** false **D.** false **E.** false

There is a high serum aminotransferases and low levels of coagulation factors such as prothrombin and factor V. Albumin and aminotransferases are not useful indicators of the course of the disease as they tend to fall along with progression of the disease.

The INR is a sensitive index of liver function and an important determinant of prognosis.

Plasma alkaline phosphatase, γ-glutamate transpeptidase, albumin and globulin concentrations are usually normal on presentation.

A 71. **A.** true **B.** true **C.** true **D.** false **E.** false

Hypokalaemic alkalosis occurs with:

- Potassium loosing diuretics
- Increased aldosterone production and mineralocorticoid drugs such as corticosteroids
- Take up into the cells with alkalosis
- Gastro-intestinal losses from vomiting and diarrhoea

Renal failure loses potassium but is associated with acidosis.

A 72. **A.** false **B.** true **C.** true **D.** true **E.** true

Transport across the placenta is not dependent on blood flow, although the amount transported may be altered.

A 73. **A.** false **B.** true **C.** false **D.** false **E.** false

The SI unit of radioactivity is the Becquerel. X-rays and γ-rays are ionising radiation because their energy is transferred into the tissue through the removal of atoms. Non-ionising radiation does not transfer atoms – such as radiowaves, infrared radiation and visible light. The rate of decay is exponential.

Infrared and radio signals have a low frequency, long wavelength and are of low energy. X-rays and γ-rays are the opposite – high energy, high frequency and short wavelength. The energy of the electromagnetic waves is proportional to the wavelength.

A 74. **A.** true **B.** true **C.** true **D.** true **E.** false

Babies are obligatory nose-breathers, so any nasal obstruction leads to breathing difficulty. TOF leads to aspiration. Diaphragmatic hernias displace lung volume.

A 75. **A.** true **B.** false **C.** false **D.** true **E.** false

HIV patients suffer from a number of opportunistic infections. The most common is *Pneumocystis carinii* pneumonia. Up to 85% of patients will develop this pneumonia at some time. It is associated with breathlessness and pyrexia. Prognosis is related to the CD4 lymphocyte cell count. A count of <100 cells per ml is associated with a poor prognosis.

A 76. **A.** true **B.** true **C.** false **D.** false **E.** false

Boyle's law, Charles's law. Vapour density is related to temperature. From Avagadro's number it is found that 1 g mol at STP occupies 22.4 l, but not at room temperature.

A 77. **A.** true **B.** false **C.** false **D.** false **E.** true

There are a number of cardiac enzymes including creatinine kinase, cardiac specific troponins, asparate aminotransferase and lactate dehydrogenase.

Troponin T and troponin I are regulatory proteins which are highly specific for cardiac injury. They are released early within 2 h of injury and can persist for up to 7 days. CK peaks in 24 h and is back to normal by 48 h. CK is also produced by damaged skeletal muscle and brain.

A 78. **A.** true **B.** true **C.** false **D.** true **E.** false

Glycine is added to saline to make the saline hypertonic. Absorption occurs but it is less than when using solutions without the glycine.

A 79. **A.** true **B.** false **C.** false **D.** true **E.** true

Student's t-test is a statistical test of parametric data. The null hypothesis proposes that there is no difference between the two groups being studied. The t-test is employed to determine the probability that any difference that is found, between two sets of results, would occur by chance.

A **80.** **A.** true **B.** true **C.** true **D.** false **E.** true

- In the first minutes after a myocardial infarction the T wave becomes tall and pointed – the ST segment is elevated
- After a few hours the T wave is inverted, the R wave voltage decreases and pathological Q waves develop
- After a few days the ST segment returns to normal
- After months the T wave may became normal again – the Q wave stays, indicating a "window" of electrical activity in the myocardium
- A pathological Q wave is >1 mm or >0.04 s and deeper than 2 mm or >0.2 mV – a Q wave can occur normally in leads AVR, V1 and III

S1, Q3, T3 is the pattern that is described in textbooks (but is rarely seen) in pulmonary embolism.

A **81.** **A.** true **B.** true **C.** false **D.** true **E.** true

The Cambridge antioxidant study found a benefit from high dose vitamin E in preventing recurrent myocardial infarction. Vitamin E is made up of tocopherols and tocotrienoles. Vitamin C and E have been used in Parkinson's disease.

A **82.** **A.** true **B.** true **C.** true **D.** true **E.** false

An epidural abscess will produce symptoms and signs by pressure on nerve roots and the spinal cord. Pain is a manifestation of nerve dysfunction. Any abnormal nerve function persisting beyond the normal period of local anaesthetic duration should be investigated.

A **83.** **A.** true **B.** true **C.** true **D.** false **E.** true

Coronary artery surgery without by-pass pumping has a large number of benefits.

A **84.** **A.** false **B.** true **C.** true **D.** true **E.** true

A 85. A. true **B.** true **C.** true **D.** false **E.** true

In obesity, the FRC is reduced mainly by a reduction in expiratory reserve volume, not residual volume.

A 86. A. true **B.** false **C.** true **D.** true **E.** true

The liver receives 1,000 ml/min of blood from the portal vein and 500 ml/min from the hepatic artery. Portal venous pressure is about 10 mmHg and the hepatic venous pressure 5 mmHg.

The hepatic veins have walls with smooth muscle supplied by noradrenergic vasoconstrictor nerves. There are no vasodilator nerves.

The only factors, which will increase hepatic blood flow are an increase in cardiac output and vasodilators of splanchnic vessels.

A 87. A. true **B.** true **C.** true **D.** true **E.** false

Aphonia may be due to damage to the vocal cords. Asphyxia can occur due to pressure on the trachea from haemorrhage into the pretracheal spaces and collapse of the trachea due to tracheomalacia. The treatment for haemorrhage is re-intubation. The blood clot can then be removed and the haemorrhage, which has usually stopped can be arrested. Tracheomalacia leading to stridor also requires re-intubation. A tracheostomy will not help as the obstruction can be low in the trachea.

Removal of the parathyroid gland may lead to hypocalcaemia and tetany.

A 88. A. false **B.** true **C.** true **D.** true **E.** false

Methyldopa is not known to be harmful. Thiazide diuretic may cause neonatal thrombocytopenia.

Isotretinion is an oral retinoid used for the treatment of acne. It carries a severe teratogenic risk if given in pregnancy. Oral anticoagulants are teratogenic and should not be given in the first trimester. They also cross the placenta and may cause foetal bleeding in the later stages of a pregnancy.

Folic acid should be given even before conception to prevent neural tube defects caused by a deficiency.

A 89. A. true **B.** false **C.** true **D.** true **E.** false

Irritable bowel syndrome is a functional disorder of the bowel with faeces containing mucus but no bleeding. Bleeding implies a disease state. There is pain and distension but no weight loss.

A 90. A. false **B.** true **C.** true **D.** true **E.** false

Red cells have no nucleus, mitochondria or ribosomes and so have limited internal functions. They cannot regenerate proteins. Energy is produced to maintain the cell membrane as a biconcave state and to keep the haemoglobin in the reduced form.
If the metabolic pathways fail the haemoglobin molecule undergoes oxidation producing methaemoglobin and globin chains inside the red cell membrane. These globin chains are called Heinz bodies. They are seen in glucose-6-phophate dehydrogenase deficiency (a failure in glucose metabolism) and haemolytic conditions with altered cell membranes.

Answers

Question	A	B	C	D	E
1	T	F	F	F	T
2	T	T	T	T	F
3	T	T	T	T	F
4	F	F	F	F	T
5	F	T	T	F	T
6	T	F	F	F	F
7	T	F	T	F	T
8	T	T	F	F	T
9	T	F	T	T	T
10	F	F	T	T	T
11	F	F	T	T	T
12	T	F	T	F	F
13	F	F	F	T	F
14	T	T	F	F	T
15	T	T	F	T	F
16	F	F	T	F	F
17	T	T	T	T	F
18	T	F	F	F	F
19	F	F	T	T	F
20	T	T	F	T	T
21	F	T	F	T	F
22	T	T	F	T	F
23	T	F	F	T	F
24	T	F	T	F	T
25	F	F	F	F	F
26	F	F	F	T	F
27	F	F	F	T	T
28	F	T	T	F	T
29	F	T	T	F	T
30	T	T	F	F	T

Question	A	B	C	D	E
31	T	T	F	F	F
32	T	T	F	F	T
33	T	F	F	T	T
34	F	F	T	F	T
35	T	T	T	F	F
36	T	F	T	F	F
37	T	T	T	F	F
38	T	T	T	T	T
39	F	F	F	F	F
40	T	T	F	F	T
41	T	T	T	F	T
42	T	T	T	F	F
43	F	T	F	T	F
44	F	F	F	F	F
45	F	T	F	F	F
46	T	F	T	T	T
47	T	T	T	T	T
48	T	F	F	F	F
49	F	F	T	F	T
50	T	F	F	F	T
51	F	F	T	F	F
52	F	F	F	T	T
53	F	F	T	F	F
54	F	T	F	T	T
55	F	T	T	F	T
56	T	T	T	F	T
57	T	T	T	T	F
58	T	T	T	F	F
59	T	F	F	F	T
60	T	T	F	T	T

Question	A	B	C	D	E
61	F	F	T	F	F
62	T	T	F	F	F
63	F	F	T	F	T
64	F	T	T	F	T
65	T	T	T	T	T
66	T	T	F	T	T
67	F	T	T	T	T
68	F	T	F	F	T
69	F	F	T	T	F
70	T	T	F	F	F
71	T	T	T	F	F
72	F	T	T	T	T
73	F	T	F	F	F
74	T	T	T	T	F
75	T	F	F	T	F
76	T	T	F	F	F
77	T	F	F	F	T
78	T	T	F	T	F
79	T	F	F	T	T
80	T	T	T	F	T
81	T	T	F	T	T
82	T	T	T	T	F
83	T	T	T	F	T
84	F	T	T	T	T
85	T	T	T	F	T
86	T	F	T	T	T
87	T	T	T	T	F
88	F	T	T	T	F
89	T	F	T	T	F
90	F	T	T	T	F

Paper 4 Answers

A 1. **A.** false **B.** true **C.** true **D.** false **E.** false

The brachial plexus arises from C5 to T1. It crosses over the first rib and lies above, behind and below the perivascular sheath.

A 2. **A.** false **B.** false **C.** true **D.** true **E.** false

Paracetamol poisoning
If gastric lavage is to be used it should only be used in the first 4 h. There is a view that gastric lavage should not be used after 1 h as it will have the effect of washing the drug further into the alimentary tract where it will be absorbed quicker.

Carbamazepine is an enzyme inducer so pre-treatment will increase the risk of liver damage.

Liver failure leads to acidosis and a prolonged PT.

Paracetamol is the most common drug used for self-poisoning.

The paracetamol is partly converted to a toxic metabolite N-acetyl-p-benzoquinolone, which is inactivated by glutathione. In an overdose, glutathione is used up and the free metabolite combines with sulphydryl groups. A series of actions leads to hepatic cell necrosis.

The antidote of choice is N-acetylcysteine. Oral methionine is an alternative but may not be possible to administer due to vomiting.

A poor prognosis is associated with an INR over 3, a pH <7.3 and a raised creatinine.

Patients with established hepatic failure might be considered for haemoperfusion or liver transplant.

The interaction of paracetamol and dextropropoxyphene with alcohol is particularly dangerous.

A 3. **A.** false **B.** false **C.** true **D.** false **E.** true

Acidosis requires a larger current. The first dose of DC reduces the resistance so the second current of 200 J is more effective than the first shock of 200 J.

A 4. **A.** false **B.** true **C.** false **D.** false **E.** false

Albumin is a polypeptide. It is synthesised in the liver and is absent from normal urine.

A 5. **A.** true **B.** true **C.** true **D.** true **E.** true

Lidocaine is a treatment for ventricular arrhythmias except after myocardial infarction.

Lidocaine, like other local anaesthetic agents, reduces the excitability of the myocardium.

A 6. **A.** false **B.** true **C.** true **D.** true **E.** false

British standard BS 4272 for oxygen warning devices
- Auditory and last for at least 7 sec
- Volume 60 db
- Powered by oxygen supply and cannot be switched off
- Alarm activated when oxygen pressure falls below 250 kPa
- The gas supply should be either progressively reduced or replaced with air as the oxygen fails

A 7. **A.** false **B.** false **C.** true **D.** false **E.** false

Hoarseness implies involvement of the recurrent laryngeal nerve. The presentation of carcinoma of the lung is usually haemoptysis. A low FEV1 is worrying but resection may remove diseased lung which is not contributing to useful lung function.

A 8. **A.** true **B.** true **C.** true **D.** true **E.** false

Any process that alters the body's ability to resist infection increases the susceptibility to sepsis.

Polycythaemia does not alter the immune state.

A 9. **A.** true **B.** false **C.** true **D.** true **E.** true

Acute asthma may lead to right heart failure and a hyper sympathetic state. The BP is increased due to hyper-sympathetic activity. The pressure required for IPPV increases the intrathoracic pressure, which normally leads to a reflex rise in central venous pressure. A high airway pressure for ventilation may lead to barotrauma of the alveoli and if the venous pressure cannot compensate the return of blood into the chest will fall.

A 10. **A.** true **B.** true **C.** true **D.** false **E.** true

Neurolept malignant syndrome occurs in a very small number of patients taking neurolepetic drugs such a haloperidol.

Symptoms include hyperthermia, muscle rigidity and autonomic dysfunction leading to tachycardias, abnormal blood pressures and variations in levels of consciousness.

Liver biochemistry is abnormal. The serum creatinine phosphokinase is raised, as is the leukocyte count.

Treatment is with bromocriptine and dantrolene to reduce muscle rigidity. General measures should protect the airway, maintain oxygenation and reduce the body temperature.

A 11. **A.** true **B.** true **C.** true **D.** false **E.** false

Most drugs are water-soluble and even if there is liver metabolism most of their elimination depends on renal excretion. Most will accumulate in renal failure. A few will quickly reach toxic levels such as opioids and digoxin.

A 12. **A.** false **B.** false **C.** true **D.** true **E.** false

It is claimed that acyclovir reduces the duration of the acute attack. It is controversial whether the incidence of post herpetic neuralgia is reduced. The problem is that a large number of patients must be treated to show a benefit in the very few patients who go on to develop post herpetic neuralgia. There is no evidence that the severity of post herpetic neuralgia, when it does occur, is less with pre-treatment with an antiviral agent.

Capsaicin is derived from peppers. It depletes the pain fibres of substance P but is painful in the first few days of treatment presumably because it is releasing substance P in the spinal cord.

Sympathetic blockade has no effect as the pain is caused by the recovery of pain fibres without the modulation of other sensory fibres.

Viruses are smaller units than micro-organisms. They contain either DNA or RNA.

DNA viruses include:

- Adenovirus
- Cytomegalo virus
- Herpes virus

A 13. **A.** true **B.** true **C.** true **D.** false **E.** false

The PCWP is greater than the LVEDP when there is an obstruction to flow into the left ventricle.

A 14. **A.** true **B.** true **C.** true **D.** false **E.** false

The blood-brain barrier is only cellular. It is more permeable in neonates. There is normally no extra cellular fluid in the brain. Lipid soluble drugs pass into the brain.

A 15. **A.** false **B.** true **C.** false **D.** true **E.** true

The femoral nerve is lateral to the artery, which is in turn lateral to the femoral vein.

The saphenous nerve is a branch of the femoral nerve.

The foot is supplied by the L4, 5 and S1 nerves roots with a large component from the sciatic nerve.

The muscles of the thigh will be affected when L2, 3 and 4 are blocked.

A 16. **A.** false **B.** false **C.** true **D.** true **E.** true

Clinically, the following tests are relevant: the sputum examined for infection or blood, the ECG for myocardial ischaemia and the PEFR for bronchospasm.

A 17. **A.** true **B.** false **C.** false **D.** true **E.** false

This question is about those scores used to assess disease severity. TISS, GCS and Ramsey scores are not about disease severity.

Paper 4

Answers

A 18. **A.** true **B.** true **C.** true **D.** true **E.** true

It is better to measure the serum creatinine than the urea as an index of renal function in the presence of normal muscle breakdown.

A 19. **A.** true **B.** true **C.** true **D.** true **E.** true

A 20. **A.** false **B.** true **C.** true **D.** true **E.** true

The pudendal nerve supplies the lower part of the vagina, the labia and with other nerves the perineum.

A 21. **A.** false **B.** true **C.** true **D.** false **E.** false

Glutamate is not classed as an essential amino acid but it is vital for normal bowel ciliary activity.

A 22. **A.** true **B.** false **C.** false **D.** false **E.** true

The TEC 3 vaporiser has a thermal control on the out flow of the gas flow. It has a larger capacity than the TEC 4. The delivered concentrations start high and gradually fall to lower levels, however efficient the temperature control.

A 23. **A.** true **B.** true **C.** true **D.** true **E.** true

Alcohol induces liver enzymes and will also produce resistance to all sedative drugs. Signs of alcoholism include raised γ-glutamyl transpeptidase, MCV $>$95 fl, carbohydrate-deficient transferrin (CDT) and HDL-cholesterol presence identify recent abuse. Blood alcohol is rarely raised at mid day while urine alcohol $>$120 mg/dl is suggestive and $>$200 mg/dl is diagnostic of chronic abuse.

Complications of alcoholism include immunosuppression, coagulation abnormalities, impaired liver function, reduced adrenocortical response to stress, peripheral or autonomic neuropathy and cardiomyopathy.

A 24. **A.** false **B.** false **C.** false **D.** true **E.** false

Pressure is measured by the Bourdon principle. The Bourdon principle can be used for temperature measurement. The flattened tube, with an ovoid cross section expands. As the tube cross section becomes more round the tube straightens and lengthens out.

A 25. **A.** true **B.** true **C.** true **D.** true **E.** true

A 26. **A.** true **B.** true **C.** false **D.** false **E.** false

Insulin requirements will be affected in renal failure if dialysis removes glucose.

Pituitary ablation will lead to an Addisonian state and β-blockers will raise the blood glucose.

A 27. **A.** true **B.** false **C.** false **D.** false **E.** false

Normal serum phosphate is 0.80 to 1.40 mmol/l. Most (80%) is within bone, while 15% is part of cell proteins such as phospholipids, nucleic acids, ATP and 2,3DPG. Hyperphosphataemia is common in chronic renal failure. Calcitonin is a polypeptide released from the thyroid gland. It antagonises parathyroid hormone and so increases calcium clearance.

A 28. **A.** false **B.** false **C.** true **D.** true **E.** false

Carboxyhaemoglobin levels are usually up to 10% in cigarette smokers and those living in a heavily smoke polluted atmosphere. Carbon monoxide has an affinity for haemoglobin about 240 times more than that of oxygen.

A 29. **A.** false **B.** true **C.** false **D.** false **E.** true

NSAIDs
The Royal College of Anaesthetists review found that NSAIDs by themselves were not enough for major surgery. There are some adults with nasal polyps who have asthma, which is made worse by NSAIDs.

A 30. **A.** false **B.** true **C.** true **D.** true **E.** false

Calcitonin is a polypeptide produced by cells in the thyroid gland. Its effects are to increase the renal excretion of calcium and phosphate and inhibit bone reabsorption. It is used in Paget's disease of bone. Parathyroid hormone is a polypeptide produced in the parathyroid glands. It increases serum calcium and reduces phosphate by increasing renal excretion.

A 31. A. false **B.** true **C.** true **D.** false **E.** true

Traumatic rupture of the thoracic aorta is more likely to occur with a blunt injury. Fracture of the upper ribs implies a severe chest injury. The presence of blood will widen the mediastinum. The oesophagus and trachea will be deviated to the right as the aorta is on the left.

A 32. A. false **B.** false **C.** false **D.** true **E.** true

MAOIs cause a rise in the resting catecholamine levels and hence abnormal blood pressures.

An epidural alone is not really suitable for upper abdominal surgery as it does not block the centre of the diaphragm or the vagus nerve. There is no protection of the airway and no control of oxygenation.

Subcutaneous heparin should be given to all major surgical cases unless there is a contraindication.

A 33. A. false **B.** true **C.** false **D.** false **E.** false

A ruptured oesophagus gives pain and surgical emphysema. Pulmonary embolism gives pain but no surgical emphysema. Rupture of the trachea or larynx gives surgical emphysema but no pain.

A spontaneous pneumothorax usually creates air in the intrapleural space around the periphery of the lung.

A 34. A. false **B.** false **C.** true **D.** false **E.** true

Hyperthyroidism is associated with:

- Cold intolerance and weight loss
- A high cardiac output and vasodilatation which will increase the pulse pressure. Tachycardia or atrial fibrillation occur
- Warm vasodilated peripheries and oligomenorrhea
- Eye signs, which include lid lag, oedema, and ophthalmoplegia

The goitre may have a bruit.

A 35. **A.** false **B.** true **C.** true **D.** false **E.** false

Tricyclic antidepressants have an anticholinergic, atropine like effect, probably through muscarinic receptors. This will lead to tachycardia and urinary retention.

They can be the cause of the central anticholinergic syndrome, which is similar to atropine intoxication. ECG changes include a longer QRS of >0.1 s, which is a predictor of arrhythmia and seizures.

A 36. **A.** true **B.** true **C.** false **D.** true **E.** true

Thiopentone has an effect of reducing cerebral metabolism and so oxygen demand. It does not alter cerebral blood flow other than by reduced vasomotor tone and reduced cardiac output.

A 37. **A.** true **B.** false **C.** false **D.** false **E.** false

Oxygen content is derived from the partial pressure of oxygen and the haemoglobin concentration. Reference is made to the oxygen dissociation curve.

Base excess is a derived value.

A 38. **A.** true **B.** true **C.** true **D.** false **E.** false

Child's grading of cirrhosis is levels A, B and C. This is based on the presence of jaundice, ascites and the level of serum albumin.

Good liver function, Child's C is:
- Albumin <30 g/l
- Bilirubin >50 Umol/l
- Ascites

Encephalopathy is important but the nutritional state is not included.

A 39. **A.** true **B.** false **C.** true **D.** false **E.** false

To perform a carotid endarterectomy the skin supplied by the roots of C3 and 4 are blocked by a deep or superficial cervical plexus block. The lesser occipital and transverse cervical nerves supply the neck. The carotid bifurcation is also blocked to prevent abnormal cardiac effects when the carotid sinus is manipulated.

A 40. **A.** true **B.** true **C.** false **D.** false **E.** true

Diamorphine is diacetylmorphine. The two acetyl molecules make it more water soluble and give it a faster onset of action and greater fat solubility, so it is better fixed in the spinal cord than morphine. Its metabolism is the same as morphine once the acetyl molecules are removed. It will give rise to M3G and M6G.

Comparable doses. Diamorphine 10 mg iv is equal to 10 mg morphine iv in the body but is often considered more potent because of the quicker speed of onset.

Morphine 10 mg is equivalent to 5 mg oxycodone, 1.5 mg hydromorphone and 100 μg of fentanyl. Equivalence of dose can vary with the route of administration and any first pass effect when given orally, or absorption if used transdermally.

A 41. **A.** false **B.** false **C.** true **D.** false **E.** false

The child is hypoxic and hypercarbic. The hypercarbia indicates an inadequate respiration. An attack of asthma starts with hyperventilation and a low carbon dioxide. When the patient becomes exhausted the carbon dioxide rises over a short period of time until death. Death can occur over the course of minutes rather than hours. This child needs urgent intubation and ventilation to give adequate oxygen, relieve the exhaustion and to facilitate the removal of thick secretion plugs. Patients die due to a failure to recognise the seriousness of exhaustion after many hours of respiratory difficulty and delay in treatment.

A 42. **A.** false **B.** true **C.** false **D.** false **E.** false

Intravenous access may further upset the child and aggravate hypoxia.

Epiglottitis is caused by *Haemophilus influenzae* usually treated with iv ceftazidine but chloramphenicol can be used. Once the proper antibiotic is given resolution only takes a day or so. Tracheostomy in small children is best avoided if at all possible.

A 43. **A.** false **B.** false **C.** false **D.** false **E.** false

Multiple sclerosis is characterised by two patterns of disease.

One form is episodes of mixed sensory and motor nerve defects which may recover partially or completely. The lesions occur in different parts of the nervous system, with no pattern.

The second form is a chronic and more progressive form affecting 25% to 30% of cases.

This disease is extremely difficult to diagnose in the early stages because it has no fixed pattern of presentation.

The eyes can be affected by blurring, loss of vision and optic neuritis. The brain stem may be affected leading to diplopia, vertigo and facial numbness. Demyelization in the spinal cord may lead to paralysis. A delayed visual evoked response follows optic neuropathy but peripheral nerves are normal.

MRI scan shows multiple plaques. The CSF can show IgG bands of immunoglobulin production in response to an unknown antigen and a raised mononuclear count.

Note that each part of this question is deceptive, as none is diagnostic.

A 44. **A.** false **B.** false **C.** true **D.** true **E.** false

The MRI is an intense magnetic field, which will affect any ferrous material.

It can interfere with pacemaker activity and older heart valves.

A 45. **A.** false **B.** true **C.** true **D.** false **E.** true

The carotid arteries supply the circle of Willis and the anterior and middle cerebral arteries with the posterior communicating arteries, within the skull. A lesion affecting the middle cerebral artery will lead to contralateral hemiplegia and hemisensory loss, facial paralysis, hemianopia and ipsilatral eye deviation.

If the dominant hemisphere is affected there will be language difficulty, aphasia or dysphasia, dysgraphia and dyscalculia. When the non-dominant side is affected it leads to neglect of the other side.

A 46. **A.** true **B.** false **C.** true **D.** false **E.** true

Constrictive pericarditis follows on from pericarditis due to tuberculous effusions, haemopericardium, bacterial infections and rheumatic heart disease. Many conditions may lead to a pericardial effusion such as uraemia but these do not lead onto a thickened pericardium.

A 47. **A.** false **B.** true **C.** false **D.** true **E.** true

Cardioplegic solutions are cold; contain potassium, magnesium, bicarbonate and dextrose. This solution leads to asystole.

Other agents that have been added include calcium channel blockers, aspartate or glutamate and adenosine regulating agents.

An alternative technique is retrograde cardioplegia via the coronary sinus. A solution of warm blood cardioplegia may be used before removal of the cross clamp on the aorta.

A 48. **A.** true **B.** false **C.** false **D.** true **E.** false

Dopexamine is an analogue of dopamine. Dopexamine is a selective β-2 agonist with less β-1 action. It also has actions on peripheral dopaminergic DA1 and DA2 receptors that may lead to better renal perfusion. It has no α-receptor action. It is a weak inotrope but it is used for its splanchnic vasodilatory effect.

Contrast this with Dobutamine, which is a β-1 agonist increasing cyclic AMP, which in turn increases myocardial contractility. Dobutamine also has an α effect leading to peripheral vasodilation. Dopamine is less selective.

Phosphodiesterase inhibitors inhibit the enzyme phosphodiesterase and reduce cyclic AMP by this mechanism.

A 49. **A.** true **B.** true **C.** false **D.** true **E.** true

HELLP syndrome is associated with haemolysis, elevated liver enzymes and low platelets.

The patient usually has an associated pre-eclampsia but not always. The APTT will usually be prolonged.

A 50. **A.** false **B.** false **C.** true **D.** false **E.** false

Verapamil
Verapamil is a class IV anti-arrhythmic. It is a calcium antagonist acting on cell membranes, which reduces the plateau phase of the action potential. These drugs slow conduction in nodal tissue.

It is indicated for use in paroxysmal supraventricular tachycardia (PSVT).

Verapamil should not be given with β-blockers or if the QRS is >0.14 s.

A 51. **A.** true **B.** true **C.** true **D.** true **E.** true

Carbon monoxide poisoning leads to:

- Hypoxia due to the formation of carboxyhaemoglobin
- Nausea and vomiting
- Headache and mental impairment
- Hallucinations, fits, drowsiness and coma

The pink colouration of the skin, due to the formation of carboxyhaemoglobin, is rarely seen before death.

Hyperbaric oxygen may be considered if the patient is pregnant, has a blood carboxyhaemoglobin over 10% and the chamber is available locally.

A 52. **A.** true **B.** true **C.** true **D.** true **E.** true

A patent foramen ovale is relatively common. The murmur is the same as that of pulmonary stenosis as more blood flows through the normal pulmonary valve.

A 53. **A.** false **B.** false **C.** true **D.** true **E.** false

The microphone is a capacitor, the thermocouple is two dissimilar plates of metal.

A 54. **A.** true **B.** false **C.** false **D.** true **E.** true

Glycolysis
Energy is stored in energy rich ATP bonds. ADP is energy depleted. Most energy is released in the Krebs cycle. The Krebs cycle releases 36 moles of ATP. Pyruvate is converted to lactate, releasing 2 ATP when there are hypoxic conditions.

A 55. **A.** true **B.** true **C.** true **D.** true **E.** true

Intra-operative bleeding will lead to hypotension and cerebral ischaemia.

A 56. **A.** true **B.** true **C.** true **D.** true **E.** true

A 57. **A.** true **B.** false **C.** true **D.** true **E.** true

TNF α, IL-6, IL-1 and granulocyte colony stimulation factor.

A 58. **A.** true **B.** false **C.** false **D.** false **E.** true

Cocaine is a local anaesthetic and vasoconstrictor. Vasoconstriction is both directed on smooth muscle and through sympathetic activity. It is a CNS stimulant. It blocks the re-uptake of dopamine. The maximum recommended dose is 1.5 mg/kg or 100 mg for an adult. The nasal spray contains 4% or 10% (40 or 100 mg/ml).

Overdose leading to tachycardia and hypertension should not be treated with β-blockers. Treatment is supportive as there is no antidote.

A 59. **A.** true **B.** true **C.** false **D.** true **E.** true

Fat embolism affects oxygenation early. Fat is seen in the circulation, the fundi and urine.

A 60. **A.** true **B.** true **C.** true **D.** false **E.** false

Haemophilia is a genetically inherited condition, linked to the male chromosome. The bleeding time (20–30 s) is the time it takes for the capillaries to contract. It is normal but the clotting time (3–5 min) is prolonged.

A 61. **A.** false **B.** true **C.** true **D.** true **E.** false

The treatment of a grand mal seizure is intravenous barbiturate, benzodiazepine, phenytoin or other anti-convulsant drug.

A 62. **A.** true **B.** true **C.** true **D.** true **E.** false

A protein load, as from the absorption of protein from the breakdown of blood in the intestine, can precipitate hepatic encephalopathy. Constipation may lead to more protein being absorbed. Barbiturates will reduce liver enzyme activity, aggravating the build-up to materials normally detoxified by the liver.

Hepatic failure can be precipitated by:

- Viruses for Hepatitis A, B, D, E
- Drugs – analgesics paracetamol, MAIO and imipramine, volatile anaesthetic halothane, anti-tuberculous isoniazid, some antiepileptics such as valproate and social drugs such as ecstasy
- Reye's syndrome, Pregnancy and Wilson's disease

A 63. **A.** false **B.** true **C.** true **D.** true **E.** true

Harrington's rods are attached to the anterior or posterior vertebral bodies joining several segments. Surgery near the spine can damage the already fragile blood supply to the cord. Open veins can lead to air embolism. The rods can enter the thoracic cage leading to a pneumothorax.

A 64. **A.** false **B.** false **C.** false **D.** true **E.** false

Isoprenaline is both an inotrope and a chronotrope. It is a peripheral vasodilator. The increased cardiac output is mostly due to an increase in heart rate. Its use is limited to heart block and severe bradycardia. Some might use it for chronic mitral regurgitation but this use is gradually declining.

A 65. **A.** true **B.** true **C.** true **D.** true **E.** true

Magnesium plasma levels are 0.7–1.1 mmol/l. An excess leads to loss of reflexes, which should be monitored during treatment. Cardiac effects include conduction defects and reduced contractility. It has a number of clinical uses including pre-eclampsia, bronchospasm and the treatment of cardiac arrhythmias.

A 66. **A.** false **B.** false **C.** false **D.** false **E.** true

The lumbar plexus is formed from roots L2 to L4. C1 carries no sensory nerves.

The lateral, and medial cutaneous nerves of the thigh supply the skin over the anterior thigh. The posterior tibial nerve is located between the medial malleolus and the Achilles tendon.

Paper 4

Answers

A 67. **A.** true **B.** false **C.** false **D.** false **E.** false

Nerve section will cause the vocal cord to be slightly abducted away from the midline. During phonation and coughing the unaffected cord, left cord, may come across the midline to meet the right cord.

A 68. **A.** false **B.** true **C.** true **D.** true **E.** false

Syntocinon causes peripheral vasodilatation with a reduction in diastolic pressure. There is likely to be a reflex tachycardia to maintain the cardiac output. If the cardiac output is maintained then systolic pressure will not fall.

Most of these effects are avoided by giving the drug slowly and in a dilute form.

A 69. **A.** true **B.** true **C.** true **D.** true **E.** true

Ulcerative colitis mostly affects the large bowel, where as Crohn's disease affects all parts of the gastrointestinal tract. Ulcerative colitis is associated with aphthous mouth ulcers.

Both inflammatory bowel diseases can be associated with:

- Eye signs of uveitis and conjunctivitis
- Gallbladder and renal stones
- Arthritis of various joints
- Liver – fatty changes
- Sclerosing cholangitis, cirrhosis, chronic hepatitis and cholangiocarcinoma
- Erythema nodosum and pyoderma gangrenosum can affect the skin

A 70. **A.** true **B.** true **C.** true **D.** true **E.** true

More serious conditions such as septic meningitis must be excluded. The 6th cranial nerve is the longest intracranial course and is often affected by disability leading to squint.

A 71. **A.** true **B.** true **C.** false **D.** false **E.** false

Thyroxine production is reduced by carbimazole and propylthiouracil. Potassium iodide 60 mg is used preoperatively to reduce gland activity and vascularity but its effect is temporary. Propranolol is used to control the effects of thyroxine but it does not reduce thyroxine levels.

A 72. **A.** false **B.** false **C.** true **D.** true **E.** true

5% glucose means 5 g in 100 ml, so there is 25 g in 500 ml.

0.5% means 0.5 g or 500 mg in 100 ml so there is 200 mg in 40 ml.

1 in 1,000 adrenaline means 1 g in 1,000 ml or 1 mg in 1 ml.

A 73. **A.** true **B.** false **C.** false **D.** true **E.** false

Digoxin toxicity occurs at >2.5 nmol/l with nausea, anorexia and altered vision, ventricular premature beats, ventricular tachycardia and AV block.

Treatment is by stopping the drug and raising potassium levels to normal. Digoxin antibodies are a specific antidote.

A 74. **A.** false **B.** false **C.** false **D.** false **E.** false

A tumour will normally have an increased blood flow compared to normal tissue.

None of these techniques is recommended.

A 75. **A.** false **B.** true **C.** false **D.** true **E.** false

It is better to treat acute conditions and improve chronic conditions before surgery. Heart failure and acute upper respiratory tract infection are better treated before elective surgery.

A 76. **A.** true **B.** true **C.** false **D.** false **E.** true

Mechanical ventilation increases the mean intrathoracic pressure. This affects cardiac output and a reflex compensation occurs causing venoconstriction in the central veins and a compensatory rise in the mean central venous pressure.

The venous return and cardiac output remain unchanged unless the patient is unable to venoconstrict or is hypovolaemic.

A 77. **A.** true **B.** false **C.** false **D.** false **E.** false

Once an infected foot is removed the demand for insulin is reduced. Acidosis is controllable because the infection is controllable and pain is reduced. Insulin requirements are reduced.

A 78. **A.** true **B.** false **C.** false **D.** false **E.** false

Cardioversion can be performed without anaesthesia in the unconscious patient. It is very painful in the awake patient.

A 79. **A.** false **B.** false **C.** true **D.** true **E.** true

DIC with a haemorrhagic state usually has a prolonged PT, PTTK and TT with low fibrinogen levels. Fibrin degradation products (FDP) are always raised. In mild cases an increase in clotting factors may maintain the PT, PTTK and TT and platelet count but the FDP will still be raised.

The skin and kidneys are most affected by thrombotic effects.

Tranexamic acid, which inhibits fibrinolysis, should not be used as it may cause a dangerous fibrin deposit. Heparin is only used as a last resort to prevent intravascular coagulation.

Fibrinolysis is a secondary response to the intravascular deposition of fibrin. It also occurs with surgery to certain tumours due to the release of tissue plasminogen activators.

A 80. **A.** true **B.** true **C.** true **D.** false **E.** true

Air embolism leads to a reduced cardiac output, which can be diagnosed as a reduction in the end tidal carbon dioxide tension but is not pathoneumonic of air embolism.

Pulmonary vascular resistance will increase as a result of obstruction or hypotensive vasoconstriction. Venous pressure will rise and increase intracranial pressure.

A 81. **A.** false **B.** false **C.** false **D.** true **E.** false

Muscle relaxation is increased by adding a muscle relaxant or increasing the effective potency of the local anaesthetic.

A 82. **A.** false **B.** false **C.** false **D.** true **E.** false

The median nerve at the elbow lies medial to the brachial muscle and tendon and medial to the brachial artery.

A 83. **A.** true **B.** false **C.** false **D.** false **E.** false

The main effect is hypoxia and acidosis followed by hypoglycaemia. The newborn has large surface area to weight, does not shiver and has a poor capacity to vasoconstrict so it loses heat easily and rapidly.

A 84. **A.** false **B.** true **C.** false **D.** false **E.** false

Vaporisers inside the circle are usually low resistance and a draw over type. In the inspiratory limb the concentration will not be diluted by adding fresh gas. The internal volume is small. Calibration is not possible and concentrations are monitored by gas analysis of inspired and expired gases. Low concentrations are used.

A 85. **A.** false **B.** true **C.** true **D.** true **E.** false

A 86. **A.** true **B.** true **C.** false **D.** true **E.** true

All anaesthetics, in low concentrations, have been associated with convulsions. Enflurane has been associated with changes in the EEG patterns.

A 87. **A.** true **B.** true **C.** true **D.** true **E.** true

A 88. **A.** true **B.** true **C.** false **D.** true **E.** false

Macrocytosis without megaloblastic changes occurs in:

- Alcohol excess, liver disease
- Reticulocytosis, hypothyroidism
- Some haematological states such as aplastic anaemia
- Cytotoxic drugs can cause it
- With cold agglutinins

An increase in reticulocytes increases the MCV because they are large cells.

Paper 4

Answers

A 89. **A.** false **B.** true **C.** false **D.** true **E.** true

Organophosphates inhibit cholinesterase and the enzyme levels will be low.

The effects are the muscarinic and nicotinic effects of acetylcholine.

- Nausea, hypersalivation
- Muscle weakness
- Bronchospasms, convulsions, respiratory failure

A 90. **A.** false **B.** false **C.** false **D.** false **E.** false

At high altitude, the number of red cells increases but not the MCHC. The oxygen dissociation curve shifts to the left.

Acclimatisation means normal oxygen delivery, so cardiac output will return to normal and airway resistance will also be normal.

Answers

Question	A	B	C	D	E
1	F	T	T	F	F
2	F	F	T	T	F
3	F	F	T	F	T
4	F	T	F	F	F
5	T	T	T	T	T
6	F	T	T	T	F
7	F	F	T	F	F
8	T	T	T	T	F
9	T	F	T	T	T
10	T	T	T	F	T
11	T	T	T	F	F
12	F	F	T	T	F
13	T	T	T	F	F
14	T	T	T	F	F
15	F	T	F	T	T
16	F	F	T	T	T
17	T	F	F	T	F
18	T	T	T	T	T
19	T	T	T	T	T
20	F	T	T	T	T
21	F	T	T	F	F
22	T	F	F	F	T
23	T	T	T	T	T
24	F	F	F	T	F
25	T	T	T	T	T
26	T	T	F	F	F
27	T	F	F	F	F
28	F	F	T	T	F
29	F	T	F	F	T
30	F	T	T	T	F

Question	A	B	C	D	E
31	F	T	T	F	T
32	F	F	F	T	T
33	F	T	F	F	F
34	F	F	T	F	T
35	F	T	T	F	F
36	T	T	F	T	T
37	T	F	F	F	F
38	T	T	T	F	F
39	T	F	T	F	F
40	T	T	F	F	T
41	F	F	T	F	F
42	F	T	F	F	F
43	F	F	F	F	F
44	F	F	T	T	F
45	F	T	T	F	T
46	T	F	T	F	T
47	F	T	F	T	T
48	T	F	F	T	F
49	T	T	F	T	T
50	F	F	T	F	F
51	T	T	T	T	T
52	T	T	T	T	T
53	F	F	T	T	F
54	T	F	F	T	T
55	T	T	T	T	T
56	T	T	T	T	T
57	T	F	T	T	T
58	T	F	F	F	T
59	T	T	F	T	T
60	T	T	T	F	F

Question	A	B	C	D	E
61	F	T	T	T	F
62	T	T	T	T	F
63	F	T	T	T	T
64	F	F	F	T	F
65	T	T	T	T	T
66	F	F	F	F	T
67	T	F	F	F	F
68	F	T	T	T	F
69	T	T	T	T	T
70	T	T	T	T	T
71	T	T	F	F	F
72	F	F	T	T	T
73	T	F	F	T	F
74	F	F	F	F	F
75	F	T	F	T	F
76	T	T	F	F	T
77	T	F	F	F	F
78	T	F	F	F	F
79	F	F	T	T	T
80	T	T	T	F	T
81	F	F	F	T	F
82	F	F	F	T	F
83	T	F	F	F	F
84	F	T	F	F	F
85	F	T	T	T	F
86	T	T	F	T	T
87	T	T	T	T	T
88	T	T	F	T	F
89	F	T	F	T	T
90	F	F	F	F	F

Paper 5 Answers

A 1. **A.** false **B.** false **C.** false **D.** false **E.** false

Autonomic dysfunction is seen but not diagnostic. The first signs are a flu like illness followed by neuromuscular weakness. CSF contains normal cell count and sugar but protein is often raised to 1 to 3 g/l. There is no evidence that steroids improve the outcome. Treatment includes IPPV, γ globulins (check for IgA deficiency first), plasmapheresis. The disease usually starts with distal muscle pain and weakness. There is reduced sensation.

Note: This is the most common acute demyelinating neuropathy. Differential diagnosis is botulism, poliomyelitis, primary muscle disease, other polyneuropathy, drug toxicity and cancer neuropathy.

A 2. **A.** false **B.** false **C.** true **D.** true **E.** true

Mortality has improved. Outcome depends on the cause not arterial gases. Trauma to the chest has a poor prognosis but fat embolism has a good prognosis. Chest X-ray shows bilateral diffuse shadowing and an air bronchogram. Hypoxaemia is a key problem as is the low compliance. One concern in treatment is not to cause barotrauma with IPPV.

A 3. **A.** true **B.** true **C.** true **D.** false **E.** true

There is usually a prolonged PT, APTT and low fibrinogen.

A 4. **A.** true **B.** true **C.** false **D.** false **E.** false

Reducing afterload involves the use of a vasodilator, nitroglycerine or sodium nitroprusside. Phentolamine will reduce venous return but tachyphylaxis develops and it is not used.

A 5. **A.** true **B.** false **C.** true **D.** true **E.** false

The body responds to a reduced renal blood flow, reduced cardiac output and increased CVP by retaining water and so increasing body water.

A 6. **A.** false **B.** false **C.** false **D.** true **E.** false

Enzyme functions tend to be poor in the newborn so it would be expected that suxamethonium will have a prolonged action. Neonates have up to 80% of their body weight as water. So they have a large extracellular volume into which the suxamethonium can dilute.

A 7. **A.** false **B.** true **C.** true **D.** false **E.** true

Bone is resorbed but there is also a compensatory increase in bone formation. The incidence increases with age. Up to 10% of adults are affected by 90 years old.

Symptoms include bone pain, most often of the spine or pelvis and deformities of tibia and cranium. Cranial nerves can be compressed leading to deafness. The cardiac output is increased to supply blood to the growing bones, resulting in heart failure. Very rarely an osteogenic sarcoma can develop.

Typical biochemistry shows a raised serum alkaline phosphatase indicating bone formation. The serum calcium and phosphate are normal with increased bone turnover.

A 8. **A.** true **B.** false **C.** true **D.** false **E.** false

The fail-safe should only depend on the falling pressure of oxygen. Some open the circuit to air but others just cut-off the nitrous oxide and close the breathing system leading to rebreathing.

A 9. **A.** false **B.** false **C.** true **D.** true **E.** true

The size of the soda lime canister is chosen to be economical.

The relief valve is positioned so that expired gas with carbon dioxide is expelled. It is inefficient to expel gas which has been "cleaned" of carbon dioxide. This position often means the circle will function like a Mapleson A and rebreathing of dead space gas will occur.

If the vaporiser is placed before the fresh gas flow the inhaled concentration will be diluted by the fresh gas flow.

A **10.** **A.** false **B.** false **C.** false **D.** true **E.** true

Tricyclic drugs are now rarely used as antidepressants but are used in the management of some neurogenic chronic pains.

Most of the effects are anticholinergic: dilated, fixed pupils and urinary retention.

Patients lose consciousness with convulsions but rarely enter into deep coma. Consciousness is regained within 24 h.

Cardiovascular effects include hypotension, tachycardia and conduction defects due to a quinine like effect. Ventricular arrhythmias are a cause of death. Most cardiac effects settle within 12 h.

Treatment is by gastric lavage and a large, single dose of activated charcoal. Gastric lavage should not be undertaken after one hour from ingestion as it may hasten absorption from the small intestine. Activated charcoal can be given at any time to slow the absorption and is not limited to 4 h.

The cardiac effects are best managed by the prevention of hypoxia. This is more important than cardiac specific drugs.

A **11.** **A.** true **B.** false **C.** false **D.** true **E.** true

Initially nitrous oxide uptake is high but being relatively insoluble a steady state is reached within minutes.

The uptake of oxygen is about 200–250 ml/min. Nitrous oxide uptake will be almost nothing after the initial minutes.

Nitrogen diffuses out of the body slower than the nitrous oxide is taken up.

A **12.** **A.** true **B.** false **C.** true **D.** false **E.** true

Urine osmolarity of 300 or equivalent to plasma implies a glomerular filtrate is reaching the bladder, diagnostic of renal tubular necrosis.

The kidney is able to conserve sodium but loses an obligatory amount of potassium.

Proteinuria implies that the renal glomerulus is allowing protein to leak out.

Creatinine is used as an index of the ability of the renal tubule to concentrate.

The normal kidney normally reabsorbs glucose.

A 13. A. false **B.** false **C.** true **D.** true **E.** true

A δ fibres transmit sharp, localised pain and C fibres transmit dull deep pain.

It uses high frequency 60–80 Hz, low intensity pulses of up to 60 mA current lasting 60–100 μs duration. In contrast acupuncture uses low frequency 5 Hz. It is thought to cause inhibition of the onward transmission of the pain stimulus in lamina II. Acupuncture has applications in the management of low intensity pains.

A 14. A. false **B.** true **C.** true **D.** false **E.** true

The oesophageal Doppler monitor measures blood flow in the arch of the aorta.

A 15. A. true **B.** false **C.** true **D.** true **E.** true

A 16. A. true **B.** true **C.** true **D.** true **E.** false

Oxygen consumption can be derived from the difference between the venous oxygen concentration and the left atrial (pulmonary artery wedge) oxygen concentration.

$SVR \times CO = BP$

The flotation catheter only goes as far as the pulmonary vein.

A 17. A. true **B.** false **C.** false **D.** false **E.** false

Thyrotoxicosis is a hypersympathetic, hypermetabolic state.

Treatment includes β-blockers, hydrocortisone, iv fluids and glucose with tepid sponge cooling if the temperature is raised.

The BNF recommends oral iodine solution, carbimazole or propylthiouracil, which may need to be given through a nasogastric tube. There is no intravenous preparation of carbimazole! This is not really an acute treatment, taking six weeks to be fully effective. Spinal anaesthesia might be appropriate but many would prefer intubation to protect the airway in a patient with gastro-intestinal obstruction.

Atropine will aggravate the tachycardia. Intravenous chlorpromazine has atropine like effects and will only act as a non-specific sedative. If cooling is required a vasodilator and tepid sponging are used.

A **18.** **A.** true **B.** false **C.** true **D.** true **E.** true

Can cause a myopathy lasting weeks and months. Myopathy seems to be associated with high doses, reduced renal function and the concurrent administration of aminoglycoside antibiotics and corticosteroids therapy. Critical care polyneuropathy is an axonal degeneration of motor and sensory nerves. The cause is not known and it is not related to muscle relaxant drugs. DVT is related to inactivity of the leg muscle pump. The paralysed patient is at risk from stretching and trauma particularly of the limbs.

A **19.** **A.** false **B.** true **C.** true **D.** true **E.** false

The age at which a routine ECG is taken without symptoms is higher than 50 – usually 65 or even higher. See NICE guidelines. Preoperative ECG should be undertaken when there are symptoms or signs or a history of cardiac disease. Chronic obstructive airway disease (COAD) may lead to a right heart disease. Anaemia should be corrected but without symptoms it is not an indication for ECG.

A **20.** **A.** true **B.** true **C.** true **D.** true **E.** true

The use of haemoglobin is about oxygen transport. 15 g/100 ml haemoglobin delivers 1,000 ml oxygen/min. Once the haemoglobin falls below 6 g/100 ml blood transfusion is recommended to maintain oxygen delivery. Patients should survive at lower levels provided they can mount an increase in cardiac output, have a proper circulation volume, are given 100% oxygen and plasma oncotic pressure is maintained.

A 21. A. true **B.** true **C.** true **D.** true **E.** false

A 22. A. true **B.** true **C.** true **D.** false **E.** true

Vertebro-basilar insufficiency affects the brain stem and posterior cortex.

It leads to dizziness, leg weakness and tetraparesis, and dysarthria or choking – also diplopia or hemianopia, vertigo and vomiting, ataxia, hemisensory loss.

In contrast, carotid insufficiency leads to cortical signs – aphasia, hemiparesis, hemisensory loss and hemianopic visual loss.

A 23. A. true **B.** true **C.** true **D.** true **E.** false

Pressure and temperature affect the density and viscosity of a gas. Similarly gas compositions will alter with changes in pressure and temperature.

A 24. A. false **B.** true **C.** true **D.** true **E.** true

Hepatitis B is caused by an incomplete DNA virus.

Hepatitis is transmitted in body fluids such as blood, semen and saliva. Transmission is usually through intravenous blood products or contaminated needles and close personal contact as in sexual intercourse. Mothers can transmit to their child at the time of birth.

Hepatitis A is transmitted by the faecal-oral route in children.

A 25. A. false **B.** true **C.** true **D.** false **E.** false

The end-tidal partial pressure of carbon dioxide must be lower than arterial $PaCO_2$ otherwise no gas will move out of the lung. Overestimation occurs as nitrous oxide is detected as carbon dioxide. They both have a molecular weight of 44. Interference can be overcome in infrared analysis by using a reference nitrous oxide cell and with the mass spectrometer by measuring a degradation product.

PEEP will enhance oxygen staying in the lung but inhibit carbon dioxide leaving the lungs.

Water vapour does not interfere with mass spectrometer measurements. It will just be measured as another gas. The molecular weight of water is 18. Infrared analysers may be affected as the total gas mixture is dried before analysis. Alveolar carbon dioxide is part of alveolar gas, which contains oxygen, nitrogen, carbon dioxide and water vapour.

A 26. **A.** true **B.** false **C.** false **D.** false **E.** false

The quick onset of action of remifentanil is due to it being less soluble than other opioids. The short duration of action is due to hydrolysis by esterases in blood and tissue but not pseudocholinesterase. It does not have an active metabolite. Half-life is 10–20 min, clearance 34 ml/kg/min. Like most opioids, it causes muscle rigidity. Most other opioids are metabolised in the liver, but elimination depends on renal excretion.

A 27. **A.** false **B.** true **C.** false **D.** false **E.** false

Ephedrine interacts with other antagonists and agonists for catecholamines. Hypertension will arise with MAOI as they increase catecholamine levels.

A 28. **A.** true **B.** true **C.** true **D.** false **E.** false

Magnesium reduces striated muscle action leading to loss of tone and reflexes. It reduces convulsions in pre-eclampsia, possibly as a result of altering blood flow.

A 29. **A.** true **B.** false **C.** true **D.** true **E.** true

Hyperbaric oxygen can be beneficial in improving oxygenation of the tissues.

Myopia is short sight.

A 30. **A.** true **B.** true **C.** true **D.** true **E.** true

Carbon monoxide is used to assess diffusion. The carbon monoxide is taken up rapidly by haemoglobin and so does not accumulate in the lung. Only 0.1% is used to prevent toxic effects of carbon monoxide. Fick's law states that: The rate of diffusion across a membrane is proportional to the concentration gradient (concentration gradient = solubility which affects the tension gradient).

Also know Graham's law – Rate of diffusion is inversely proportional to the square root of molecular weight.

Liquids diffuse less rapidly than gases.

A 31. **A.** true **B.** true **C.** true **D.** false **E.** false

Low sodium, high potassium is explained by renal tubular disease, reduced mineralocorticoids in Addison's disease and hypopituitary states.

Hyperaldersteronism will raise the sodium, lower potassium and raise BP as occurs in Cushing's disease.

Make a list of the causes of high and low sodium, high and low potassium.

A 32. **A.** true **B.** false **C.** true **D.** true **E.** true

Intraocular pressure will rise with hypoxia and other states that increase catecholamines.

A 33. **A.** false **B.** false **C.** true **D.** false **E.** true

Mitral stenosis is associated with:

Palpation – an apex beat which is tapping – palpable first heart sound and right ventricular enlargement but the apex beat is not displaced (as with an enlarged left ventricle). There will be a palpable thrill with tricuspid incompetence.

Auscultation – the first heart sound is accentuated if the valve is pliable. The valve opens with an opening snap after the second sound. There is a mid diastolic murmur with pre-systolic accentuation.

The severity of the stenosis can be judged by the presence of pulmonary hypertension and right heart strain, which leads to pulmonary incompetence. Stenosis is more severe when the opening snap is close to the second sound and the mid-diastolic murmur is longer.

Paper 5 Answers

A 34. **A.** true **B.** true **C.** true **D.** false **E.** false

Radial nerve innervates the extensor of the wrist and fingers. It curves round the humerus where it is injured by pressure. Saturday night palsy is caused by the drunk with his arm over the back of the chair putting pressure on the radial nerve as it curves round the humerus.

Elbow extension is mediated by the triceps muscle.

The base of the thumb is supplied by the median nerve.

The radial nerve supplies brachioradialis not pronator teres.

A 35. **A.** true **B.** true **C.** true **D.** true **E.** true

Pulmonary embolism is associated with breathlessness and chest pain. Right heart strain and raised CVP. Initially there is a hyperadrenergic state until lung blood flow is obstructed and then cardiac output falls.

A 36. **A.** true **B.** true **C.** true **D.** false **E.** true

Herpes zoster is caused by a DNA virus similar to the chicken pox virus. The infection affects all diameter fibres but the large diameter fibres are the last to return to function, hence pain transmitted by the small diameter fibres.

A 37. **A.** true **B.** true **C.** false **D.** true **E.** true

Do not confuse ropivacaine with laevobupivacaine, the isomer of bupivacaine. Cardiac side effects are less likely.

A 38. **A.** true **B.** true **C.** true **D.** true **E.** true

Amiodarone increases the refractory period of cardiac muscle and so inhibits atrial and ventricular re-entry rhythms. Long plasma half-life of 10 to 100 days.

Side effects include reduced vision due to corneal opacities and night glare, hypothyroidism, peripheral neuropathy and myopathy and gastrointestinal disturbances. Photosensitivity may rarely lead to a slate grey skin.

A 39. **A.** true **B.** false **C.** false **D.** true **E.** false

The effects of altitude include:

Reduced atmospheric oxygen tension – at 3,000 m, alveolar oxygen will be 8 kPa (60 mmHg). The alveolar tension of oxygen falls rapidly (alveolar air equation) as alveolar carbon dioxide tensions falls only a little and water vapour tension remains constant. (Contrast with what happens to alveolar gases in the non-breathing patient in recovery.)

Low arterial oxygen tensions leads to vasodilatation, which may lead to increased capillary pressure and transudation of fluid into cerebral tissue.

Pulmonary vasoconstriction due to lung hypoxia leads to pulmonary hypertension.

Erythropoietin secretion increases to increase the red cells mass and PCV, but no increase in plasma volume.

Initially the patient has a mild ventilatory response as the alkalosis counteracts the hypoxia effect. In time, ventilation increases due to active transport of hydrogen ions into the CSF or there is a lactic acidosis.

A 40. **A.** true **B.** false **C.** false **D.** false **E.** true

α-blockers cause vasodilatation, which will reduce blood pressure and lead to postural hypotension.

A 41. **A.** true **B.** true **C.** false **D.** false **E.** false

Cyanotic heart disease is due to venous blood entering the systemic circulation having by passed the lung. This can occur through an abnormal passage as in Fallot's tetralogy and transposition of the great vessels. In other conditions pulmonary hypertension must develop to reverse the normal left to right shunt.

A 42. **A.** true **B.** true **C.** true **D.** false **E.** false

Anti-D antibodies develop when blood from an Rh-positive foetus mixes with blood from an Rh-negative mother. This can occur any time in pregnancy including during miscarriages and terminations.

Paper 5 Answers

A 43. **A.** true **B.** true **C.** true **D.** true **E.** true

A 44. **A.** false **B.** false **C.** true **D.** true **E.** false

Polymyalgia rheumatica is a systemic disease of the elderly. Myopathy by itself means weak muscles but not painful muscles. The rheumatica plus myopathy means there is sudden onset of proximal, morning pain and stiffness. Diagnosis is associated with a raised ESR and CRP and anaemia. 10–30% have an associated giant cell arteritis.

A 45. **A.** false **B.** false **C.** true **D.** false **E.** false

Tetanus can be present in four forms:

- *Generalised* – has a poor prognosis, short incubation period and a short onset phase – that is the period from symptoms of being unwell to the onset of spasms – usually 1–3 days. The shorter incubation and the shorter the onset period the poorer is the prognosis
- *Localised* – with local muscle spasms
- *Cephalic* – often from a middle ear infection – usually fatal
- *Neonatal* – from an umbilical infection – usually fatal

Mortality in general tetanus rises with:

- Extremes of age
- Short incubation period
- Short interval from symptoms to spasms
- iv opioid drug addicts

Immunity needs to be boosted by regular immunisation.

A 46. **A.** false **B.** false **C.** false **D.** true **E.** true

Plummer-Vincent syndrome is a web in the upper oesophagus associated with glossitis and angular stomatitis. It affects women more than men. It is of unknown origin but associated with iron deficiency anaemia.

A 47. **A.** true **B.** true **C.** true **D.** false **E.** false

Aprotinin inhibits proteolytic enzymes such as plasmin and kallidinogens (kallikrein). It is also used to inhibit hyperplasminaemia found in some tumours associated with acute promyelocytic leukaemia.

Rare side effects include hypersensitivity and thrombophlebitits.

It is given until bleeding stops in major heart surgery, liver surgery and major blood loss.

A 48. **A.** false **B.** true **C.** false **D.** false **E.** true

In sickle cell disease, the Hb is usually 6–8 g/dl. There is no HbA but 80–90% HbS and up to 20% HbF.

Splenic infarcts lead to a small spleen. The patients are not iron deficient. Sickle cell crises are precipitated by hypoxia during anaesthesia and high altitudes.

Sickle trait has 60% HbA and 40% HbS.

A 49. **A.** false **B.** false **C.** true **D.** false **E.** false

The lateral cutaneous nerve of the forearm, which comes from the musculo-cutaneous nerve, supplies the lateral forearm.

A 50. **A.** true **B.** true **C.** true **D.** true **E.** true

A 51. **A.** true **B.** true **C.** true **D.** true **E.** true

Parkinson's disease is associated with heartburn, dysphagia, constipation and weight loss. Dysphagia may lead to regurgitation.

Arrhythmias have been reported with high doses of levodopa. Levodopa may lead to a reduced intravascular volume and postural hypotension.

Upper airway muscles can be affected by the extrapyramidal disorder leading to airway obstruction and abnormal flow-volume loops. Autonomic dysfunction can occur as the disease advances. Phenothiazines can aggravate extrapyramidal symptoms.

A 52. **A.** false **B.** true **C.** true **D.** false **E.** false

Antithrombin III is a blood product used to treat congenital factor AT III deficiencies. It is an α-2 globulin.

The clotting cascade is slowed by a number of inhibitors. One of the most important inhibitors is antithrombin III. It neutralises thrombin and all the serine proteases in the cascade Xa, IXa, XIa and XIIa.

Other inhibitors are:

- Heparin co-factor II, which blocks only thrombin
- Heparin sulphate and heparin are released from the endothelium
- α-2 macroglobulin and α-2 anti-trypsin
- C1 activator inhibits the complement cascade and some coagulation factors – a deficiency of C1 increases the risk of thromboembolism

A **53.** **A.** true **B.** true **C.** true **D.** true **E.** true

A **54.** **A.** false **B.** true **C.** true **D.** false **E.** false

Neisseria are gram-negative diplococci.

There are only two – meningitides and gonorrhoea that are pathogenic to humans.

Group A is common in Africa and Group B in Europe and America. C, Y and W135 are increasing worldwide.

Treatment should start with benzylpenicillin 1.2–2.4 g iv four hourly. Cefotaxime dose starts at 50 mg/kg and in severe infections increases to 200 mg/kg in children. In adults 6 g/day or 100 mg/kg. Treatment is usually continued for 5–7 days to avoid resistant strains.

A **55.** **A.** true **B.** false **C.** false **D.** false **E.** true

Gabapentine is an adjunctive drug for partial seizures. It has recently been used in the control of neurogenic pain. It can cause sedation and other central nervous disturbances such as tremor and diplopia. Also nausea and vomiting, but it is well tolerated by most people. There is a suggestion of a threshold dose at about 1.8 g.

Despite its name it has as no relationship to GABA receptors.

Antacids reduce absorption, otherwise it is free of interactions.

A **56.** **A.** true **B.** true **C.** true **D.** false **E.** false

Cytokines that have immunoregulatory action include tumour necrosis factor (TNF), lymphotoxins and interferon-γ (IFN-γ).

The nature of the immune response is regulated by cytokines. Type 1 help or immune response produced by Interleukin-2 (IL-2) and IL-12 and IFN- γ. A type 2 help or antibody-mediated response induced by IL-4, IL-6 and IL-10.

A **57.** **A.** true **B.** false **C.** false **D.** true **E.** false

Mivacurium is a short acting, non-depolarising muscle relaxant metabolised by pseudocholinesterase. The amount of histamine released depends on the speed of injection, displacing histamine from the mast cells.

A **58.** **A.** false **B.** true **C.** true **D.** false **E.** false

Paramagnetic analysers analyse paramagnetic gases. Oxygen and nitric oxide are the only two paramagnetic gases of clinical significance. The analyser needs calibration but is then very stable and reliable with a long life. The downside is that they are expensive.

A **59.** **A.** false **B.** true **C.** false **D.** true **E.** false

One problem for patients with aortic stenosis is that symptoms appear late in the disease. Sudden death can be the first sign. The hypertrophied myocardium is vulnerable to ischaemia. An increase in heart rate reduces the time for coronary filling. Reducing the heart rate will allow more coronary blood flow.

A higher inspired oxygen tension increases the oxygen gradient to the tissues.

The stenosis means that cardiac output is limited. Any measure that causes vasodilatation may drop the blood pressure if the cardiac output cannot be increased enough.

A **60.** **A.** true **B.** false **C.** false **D.** false **E.** false

Pregnancy is associated with lower CSF volume and a smaller epidural space with larger epidural veins.

A **61.** **A.** false **B.** true **C.** false **D.** true **E.** false

Lithium is used to treat mania and manic-depressive disorders. It substitutes for sodium and potassium and so affects many metabolic pathways.

Paper 5

Answers

Long term use is associated with hypothyroid disease, memory impairment, fine tremor, inhibition of ADH leading to polydipsia, increased appetite and weight gain. There is a narrow therapeutic/toxic ratio with a therapeutic serum level <1.5 mmol/l.

The effect of lithium is potentiated by low serum sodium concentrations.

It should be stopped two days pre-operatively with fluid and electrolyte monitoring. It has many interactions. There is reduced excretion with NSAIDs and the effect of muscle relaxants is enhanced.

A **62. A.** false **B.** true **C.** true **D.** true **E.** false

Halothane breaks down to give fluoride ions.

A **63. A.** true **B.** false **C.** true **D.** true **E.** true

Bleeding will be increased by increased BP and cardiac output as occurs with any increase in sympathetic activity due to hypoxia, pain, and over transfusion. High venous pressure will increase venous bleeding.

A **64. A.** false **B.** true **C.** false **D.** true **E.** false

Brain stem death diagnosis has specific criteria:

- The serum chemistry must be normal for electrolytes, glucose
- There should be no effect from analgesics, muscle relaxants or sedatives
- Normal temperature and arterial blood gases

The tests are for reflexes of the cranial nerves and apnoea at normal carbon dioxide tensions with no hypoxia. Peripheral muscle movement and spinal cord reflexes may occur.

A **65. A.** true **B.** false **C.** false **D.** false **E.** true

IPPV increases the mean intrathoracic pressure and the mean central venous pressure must also rise to maintain venous return into the thorax. Lung physiology is altered. There is long term retention of salt and water and an increased risk of infection.

A 66. A. false **B.** false **C.** true **D.** false **E.** true

Aminoglycosides are nephrotoxic and not ideal for chest infections.

Anaemia is usually present in severe cases as is pruritus due to the retention of nitrogenous waste.

The gastro-intestinal tract is affected by delayed gastric emptying, peptic ulceration, risk of pancreatitis and constipation. Gout due to urate retention and raised cholesterol and triglycerides is common.

There are various changes in endocrine levels, some as a result of lower protein binding. LH is raised, testosterone low, growth hormone low, thyroid hormones usually low and calcium is raised with an associated hyperparathyroidism. The heart may suffer from hypertension and pericarditis.

If fluid and electrolyte balance is normal and there is no renal ischaemia, BP will be normal.

Suxamethonium will lead to a rise on serum potassium of 0.5 mmol/l. This is only a problem if the serum potassium is already high.

A 67. A. false **B.** false **C.** false **D.** false **E.** true

Helium has been recommended for turbulent upper airway obstruction but the cylinder is normally supplied with 21% oxygen and 79% helium at a time when most anaesthetists would want to give higher concentrations of oxygen. Helium is less dense that nitrogen. Turbulent flow is proportional to density. Normally the smaller airways have laminar flow and helium would make no difference.

A 68. A. true **B.** false **C.** true **D.** true **E.** true

The lung is ventilated but not perfused, surfactant is no longer produced by non-perfused lung and alveolar collapse occurs.

Chest X-ray is often normal but linear atelectasis or small pleural effusion may be seen. After some time a raised hemi diaphragm and a wedge where the pulmonary artery flow is cut off is seen.

ECG shows right ventricular strain.

If cardiac output drops the patient may suffer from syncope attacks.

D-dimer levels
Plasmin – a serum protease – breaks down fibrinogen and fibrin into fragments or fibrin degradation products. Cross-linked fibrin gives D-dimer and D-dimer fragments. Absence of plasma D-dimer excludes pulmonary embolism. A raised level supports but does not confirm a diagnosis.

A 69. **A.** true **B.** false **C.** true **D.** false **E.** false

Gas chromatography is used to analyse mixtures of volatile agents and is good for small concentrations and mixtures of gases with liquids.

There is no Raman scattering. It is the Raman spectrometry. When light acts on a gas molecule the energy of the molecule changes. The light either gives up or receives energy, which alters the wavelength of the gas. The change in wavelength is characteristic of each gas molecule. This is called the Raman effect.

A 70. **A.** true **B.** true **C.** false **D.** false **E.** false

This lady is dehydrated with fluid and electrolyte loss.

The tachypnoea indicates hypoxia and the hypotension shows a low cardiac output. She will be oliguria and then uraemia.

Her liver store of glycogen will be low so she may be hypoglycaemic.

A 71. **A.** false **B.** true **C.** false **D.** false **E.** true

The first line treatment is to look for a cause, e.g. hypoxia, hypercarbia, dehydration.

The drugs of choice are amiodarone or lidocaine.

A 72. **A.** false **B.** false **C.** false **D.** true **E.** false

Local anaesthetic to the pyriform fossa produces a superior laryngeal nerve block.

A 73. **A.** false **B.** true **C.** true **D.** false **E.** false

The two ways of assessing oxygen concentrations in theatre are either by using a fuel cell or by the use of paramagnetic analyser. The oxygen electrode is used in laboratories for blood analysis. The fuel cell has a membrane that allows oxygen to diffuse through and dissolve into a solution. This then creates a battery and a current. The fuel cell and the oxygen electrode use the same principle in which oxygen combines with electrons and water to form hydroxyl ions. This process is oxidation as it adds oxygen. Oxidation releases energy, which is the basis for the production of the current.

The paramagnetic property of oxygen means that it is drawn into a magnetic field. The only other clinically used paramagnetic gas is nitric oxide.

A 74. **A.** true **B.** false **C.** true **D.** false **E.** false

It is always appropriate to increase the inspired oxygen. The implication is that the patient has a tension pneumothorax or cardiac tamponade due to blood in the pericardial sac.

A chest drain would be indicated for the pneumothorax. IPPV would increase the tension pressure.

A 75. **A.** true **B.** true **C.** true **D.** true **E.** true

Venous thromo-embolism causes a reduction in blood flow through the lungs and hence a reduced cardiac output.

Arrhythmias will occur. The end tidal CO_2 is reduced if cardiac output falls.

A 76. **A.** true **B.** true **C.** false **D.** true **E.** false

Polycystic renal disease is an autosomal dominant condition. About 30% of cases have hepatic cysts.

It presents from teenage onwards with loin pain and haematuria. 8% have a berry aneurysm leading to a subarachnoid haemorrhage. There may be hypertension, uraemia and anaemia and complications of the cysts.

Survival rates with regular dialysis are similar to other renal diseases.

Patients can be offered the full range of dialysis and renal transplantation.

A 77. **A.** true **B.** true **C.** false **D.** true **E.** false

Increased heart rate and hypertension implies an excess of sympathetic activity due to a surgical stimulus or hypercarbia, or an over filled circulation will occur with a hyper-osmolar state.

A 78. **A.** true **B.** false **C.** false **D.** false **E.** true

Acute atrial fibrillation is treated with electrical cardioversion and attention to the cause. Heart block can be treated with epinephrine or isoprenaline, or pacing, depending on the cause and cardiac output.

A 79. **A.** false **B.** false **C.** false **D.** true **E.** true

Pressure gauges measure gas pressure in kPa and less frequently in psi and bars. They do not reduce pressures.

A 80. **A.** true **B.** false **C.** false **D.** true **E.** false

The EMO has an expanding bellows to control the temperature compensation.

Temperature compensation in a Mark II, III and IV vaporiser is by a bimetallic strip. This strip is within the vaporising chamber, controlling the gas coming in rather than on the outlet.

The Dräger vapouriser has an expansion sensor on the outlet. The miniature Oxford vaporiser is not temperature compensated. Penlon vaporisers have a bellows within the chamber.

A 81. **A.** false **B.** true **C.** true **D.** true **E.** true

Malignant hypothermia is an inherited, congenital defect in which calcium ions, once taken up are not released and contraction continues.

ATPase activity is impaired and the intracellular pH falls as the cells become more hypoxic.

A **82.** **A.** true **B.** true **C.** true **D.** false **E.** false

Calcified coronary vessels make surgery difficult.

A **83.** **A.** true **B.** true **C.** false **D.** true **E.** false

Electrical frequencies in the region of 50 Hz are most likely to induce ventricular arrhythmias in the heart. Diathermy frequencies are much higher at 1 MHz.

Current density is highest at the point of entry to the body to cause a heating effect.

A **84.** **A.** false **B.** false **C.** true **D.** true **E.** false

The stoichiometric concentration of a mixture is the concentration at which all the combustible vapour is used up. Pure oxygen under pressure is a high explosion risk.

Plastic burns better than rubber.

A **85.** **A.** false **B.** true **C.** false **D.** false **E.** true

Peptic ulceration is aggravated by NSAIDs but not by paracetamol. Curling's ulcers are associated with burns and occur in the stomach, not in the duodenum. *Helicobacter pylori* are identified as a causative agent in many cases of peptic ulceration.

A **86.** **A.** true **B.** false **C.** true **D.** true **E.** false

Liver transplants are unlikely to be performed on patients with normal liver enzyme function. The patient needs to be as well as possible. This includes good renal function, control of nitrogen balance and ascites.

A **87.** **A.** true **B.** false **C.** true **D.** true **E.** false

Parasympathetic nerves link to the III, VII, IX and X cranial nerves.

A **88.** **A.** true **B.** true **C.** true **D.** true **E.** false

Calcification on chest X-ray can be seen with asbestosis, calcified valves and lymph nodes.

A **89.** **A.** true **B.** false **C.** true **D.** false **E.** false

In WPW syndrome, digoxin should not be given as it may slow the normal sinus node and encourage re-entry of the abnormal impulses.

A **90.** **A.** true **B.** false **C.** false **D.** true **E.** true

Polymorpho-nuclear leukocytes are seen in response to an infecting organism.

A rise in a mixed picture of polymorphs and lymphocytes may be seen in meningitis due to viruses, neoplasms, infection in arteries or veins, after subarachnoid haemorrhage, and rarer conditions such as cerebral malaria, sarcoidosis and Lyme's disease.

Answers

Question	A	B	C	D	E
1	F	F	F	F	F
2	F	F	T	T	T
3	T	T	T	F	T
4	T	T	F	F	F
5	T	F	T	T	F
6	F	F	F	T	F
7	F	T	T	F	T
8	T	F	T	F	F
9	F	F	T	T	T
10	F	F	F	T	T
11	T	F	F	T	T
12	T	F	T	F	T
13	F	F	T	T	T
14	F	T	T	F	T
15	T	F	T	T	T
16	T	T	T	T	F
17	T	F	F	F	F
18	T	F	T	T	T
19	F	T	T	T	F
20	T	T	T	T	T
21	T	T	T	T	F
22	T	T	T	F	T
23	T	T	T	T	F
24	F	T	T	T	T
25	F	T	T	F	F
26	T	F	F	F	F
27	F	T	F	F	F
28	T	T	T	F	F
29	T	F	T	T	T
30	T	T	T	T	T

Paper 5 Answers

Question	A	B	C	D	E
31	T	T	T	F	F
32	T	F	T	T	T
33	F	F	T	F	T
34	T	T	T	F	F
35	T	T	T	T	T
36	T	T	T	F	T
37	T	T	F	T	T
38	T	T	T	T	T
39	T	F	F	T	F
40	T	F	F	F	T
41	T	T	F	F	F
42	T	T	T	F	F
43	T	T	T	T	T
44	F	F	T	T	F
45	F	F	T	F	F
46	F	F	F	T	T
47	T	T	T	F	F
48	F	T	F	F	T
49	F	F	T	F	F
50	T	T	T	T	T
51	T	T	T	T	T
52	F	T	T	F	F
53	T	T	T	T	T
54	F	T	T	F	F
55	T	F	F	F	T
56	T	T	T	F	F
57	T	F	F	T	F
58	F	T	T	F	F
59	F	T	F	T	F
60	T	F	F	F	F

Question	A	B	C	D	E
61	F	T	F	T	F
62	F	T	T	T	F
63	T	F	T	T	T
64	F	T	F	T	F
65	T	F	F	F	T
66	F	F	T	F	T
67	F	F	F	F	T
68	T	F	T	T	T
69	T	F	T	F	F
70	T	T	F	F	F
71	F	T	F	F	T
72	F	F	F	T	F
73	F	T	T	F	F
74	T	F	T	F	F
75	T	T	T	T	T
76	T	T	F	T	F
77	T	T	F	T	F
78	T	F	F	F	T
79	F	F	F	T	T
80	T	F	F	T	F
81	F	T	T	T	T
82	T	T	T	F	F
83	T	T	F	T	F
84	F	F	T	T	F
85	F	T	F	F	T
86	T	F	T	T	F
87	T	F	T	T	F
88	T	T	T	T	F
89	T	F	T	F	F
90	T	F	F	T	T